28
DAYS
to
Gut
health

Clémence Cleave & Giovanna Torrico
Photography by Lisa Linder

28 DAYS *to* Gut **health**

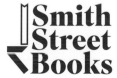

Smith
Street
Books

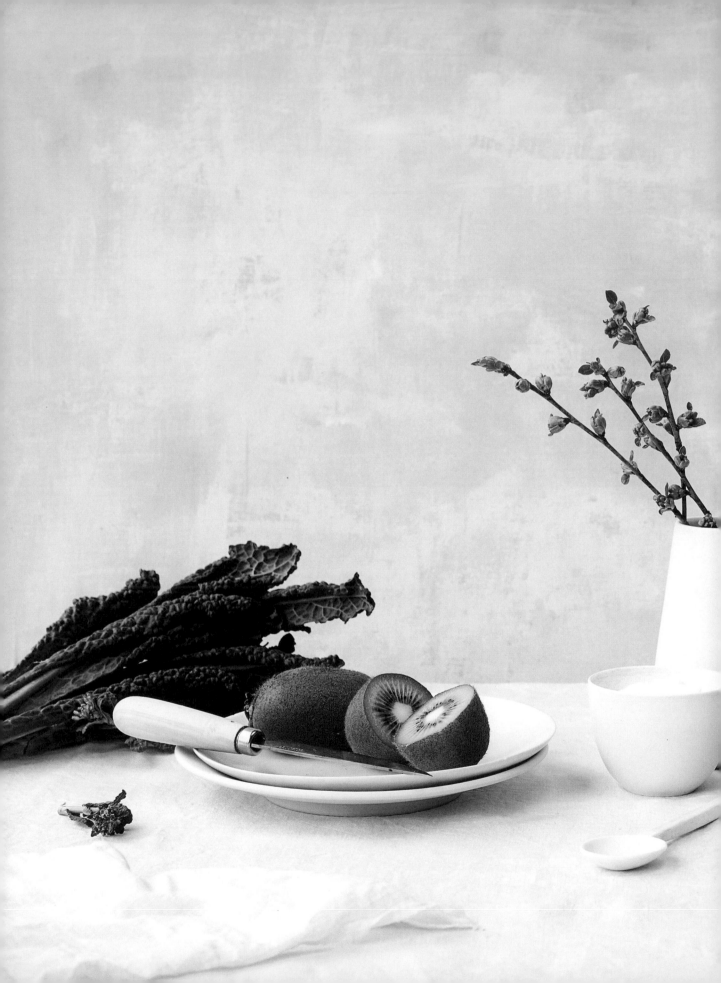

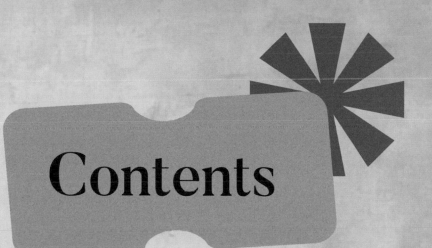

Contents

Why Gut Health
Matters?

Have you ever had a gut feeling? Do you sometimes feel gutted? Or even gutsy? Instinctively, we have always known that the gut is more than just a digestive tube. Scientists even call it our second brain. But what's so unique about our gut and why does it matter?

The gut is at the core of well-being. Obviously, it is first and foremost the site where your digestion and nutrition happen: the food you eat is churned, broken down, absorbed, transformed and moved down the digestive tract to feed the body. But recent discoveries reveal that the gut plays many more roles in health and well-being: it interacts with your immune functions, communicates with your brain, affects your mood and regulates your energy levels and appetite. It is a fascinating system that is influenced by what you eat, your environment and your behaviour.

1 The large intestine – not so stinky after all

It is easy to underestimate the large intestine (aka the colon). Long regarded as just a place for undigested food waste to linger before being pooped out, it is home to ill-smelling gases, an unpredictable appendix and more-or-less regular bowel movements – nothing very sexy. Then, in the 19th century, the concept of gut flora emerged. Scientists discovered that the gut was host to multiple microorganisms, some associated with good health, others with illness. But it is only in the last two decades, with the rise of genetic sequencing technology that scientists have started to realise the key roles that this internal ecosystem plays.

2 Busy microbes

Although the gut is inside you, it is actually an external organ, acting as the primary gateway into your body. With up to 1.8 kg (4 lb) of

food eaten every day, there are lots of 'foreign' compounds trying to enter this portal. A bit like the door staff of a club, you need a reliable system to check what can safely be let in and what needs to be kept out. The gut microbes act as busy bouncers, making a physical barrier and constantly liaising with management (your brain) to protect you from undesirable visitors.

3 When things go wrong

Unfortunately, things can go wrong. If the gut microbiota is damaged – with the use of alcohol or antibiotics, for example, or with factors beyond our control – these lines of defence get weakened. Thankfully this is usually only temporary but in some cases, it can lead to chronic disorders or diseases (e.g. allergic reactions, lupus, Coeliac disease, Crohn's disease, ulcerative colitis).

4 Take care of your gut microbiota

By nourishing and protecting your gut microbiota you can support your health and well-being. And what you eat matters: choosing a diet with lots of plant-based food rich in dietary fibre, polyphenols and fermented foods will help the gut microbiota flourish and thrive. Other aspects of life will also affect the gut microbiota: pollution, stress, medication, physical activity and sleep. In this book you will find lots of tasty recipes and useful health habits for taking care of your 'second brain'.

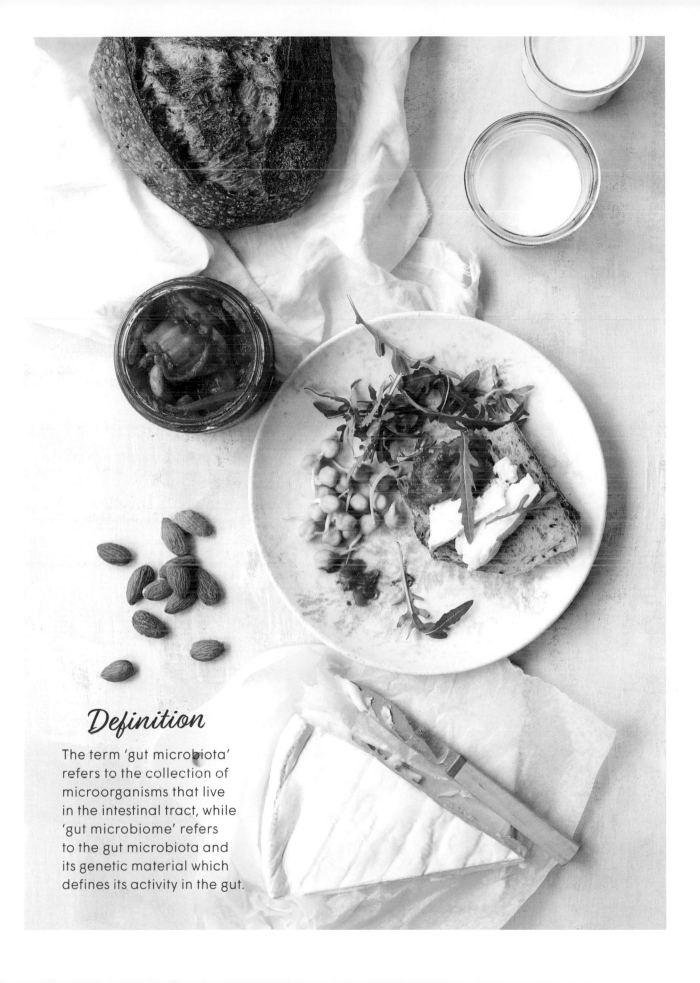

Definition

The term 'gut microbiota' refers to the collection of microorganisms that live in the intestinal tract, while 'gut microbiome' refers to the gut microbiota and its genetic material which defines its activity in the gut.

Understanding
Your Gut

Your digestive tract, aka the gut, is central to your body, literally.
It is 6 metres (20 feet) long, starting from the mouth and finishing with the
anus. The food you eat will take up to 72 hours to complete its journey
through the gut, during which a lot of action will take place.

1 Digestion

It all starts in the mouth. Food gets broken down through actions both mechanical (by chewing and churning) and chemical (with enzyme and acid release) as it travels through the oesophagus, the stomach and the small intestine.

→ Carbohydrates are transformed into simple sugar molecules.

→ Proteins are turned into small amino acids.

→ Fats are dispersed into tiny droplets.

→ Minerals and vitamins are set free, floating into the digestive tract.

This process is essential: it extracts the nutrients (ready for absorption) from the food, while the other food components can carry on their journey and finally get pooped out.

2 Absorption

It is in the small intestine that most of the absorption happens. Here, broken-down food makes its way through 3–5 metres (10–16 feet) of tube with lots of folds covered in hair-like projections, called microvilli (a bit like a sea anemone) to increase its surface area and give more chance for nutrients to get across the gut wall into the body. Glucose molecules, amino acids and other water-soluble nutrients (some vitamins and minerals) join the bloodstream, while droplets of fats and vitamins A, D, E and K join the lymphatic system. After 2–6 hours, any unabsorbed nutrients and undigested food move further on, into the large intestine.

3 In the large intestine

Here, things slow right down – it can take more than two days for the food to travel only 1.5 metres (5 feet). And here is where some true magic happens. The microorganisms that live in the large intestine start feasting on the food that hasn't been digested, releasing lots of compounds called metabolites (page 16):

→ B vitamins and vitamin K that then get absorbed

→ molecules that act as strong signals to the brain.

LIKE A DOUGHNUT!

Did you know that your gastrointestinal tract is in fact external to you? It is a long tube surrounded by the body in which food travels and gets churned, broken down, assimilated or discarded. Some have even compared the body to a doughnut where the gastrointestinal tract would be the hole in the middle.

The digestive system

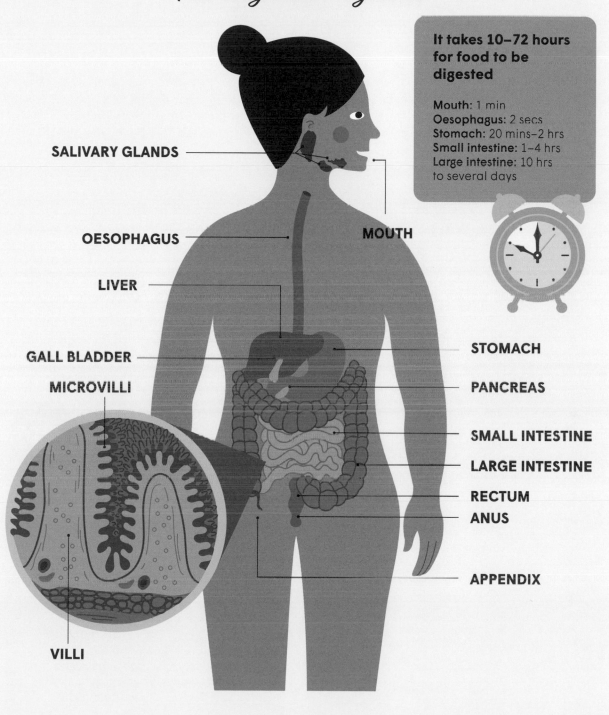

It takes 10–72 hours for food to be digested

Mouth: 1 min
Oesophagus: 2 secs
Stomach: 20 mins–2 hrs
Small intestine: 1–4 hrs
Large intestine: 10 hrs to several days

SALIVARY GLANDS

MOUTH

OESOPHAGUS

LIVER

STOMACH

GALL BLADDER

PANCREAS

MICROVILLI

SMALL INTESTINE

LARGE INTESTINE

RECTUM

ANUS

APPENDIX

VILLI

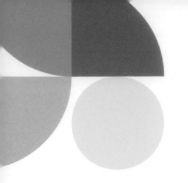
Powerful
Signalling

What goes on in the digestive tract affects the whole body. If the brain is command HQ, the gut is the secret intelligence that reports back, informing on the need for action from other organs. You should really trust your gut!

1 Communication lines

The gut is constantly sending all kinds of signals via three main channels:

→ your nervous system

→ your immune system

→ your blood circulatory system.

Those signals target many organs: brain, liver, fat tissues, lungs, skin and muscles – all of which respond to the messages.

2 Appetite …

When the body needs energy but energy stores are down and the gut is empty, it sends a hormonal signal to the brain saying, 'it is time to eat'. When food is ingested and detected in the stomach, it sends a nerve signal to say, 'it feels like we are eating, nutrients coming soon!', which reassures the brain. And when nutrients finally reach the small intestine, satiety hormones are released saying to the brain and the liver, 'it looks like we have enough energy to sustain us for a while' – and this switches off your appetite.

3 … and beyond

The gut sends many signals that influence other aspects of your health. For example, it warns when the body is besieged by harmful pathogens and it informs your immune system about how hard it needs to fight back. It also modulates your experience of pain and sharpens your cognitive functions. It influences the levels of cholesterol in your bloodstream, it modulates your sensitivity to insulin and it affects your body fat accumulation.

Talkative microbes

It is the gut microbiota that is responsible for triggering and modulating many of these signals. Your colony of microbes stimulates the secretion of hormones (e.g. controlling hunger and satiety) and neurotransmitters (e.g. dopamine or serotonin). It can also prompt an immune response or an inflammation (e.g. skin rash) or send stress signals to the brain.

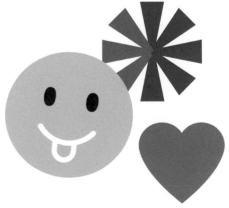

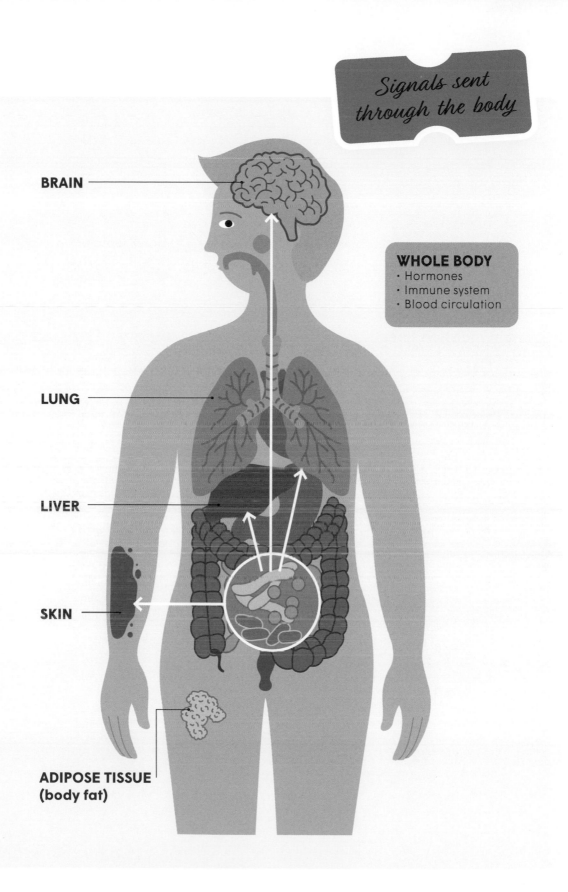

BRAIN

LUNG

LIVER

SKIN

ADIPOSE TISSUE
(body fat)

WHOLE BODY
· Hormones
· Immune system
· Blood circulation

Inside the intestines

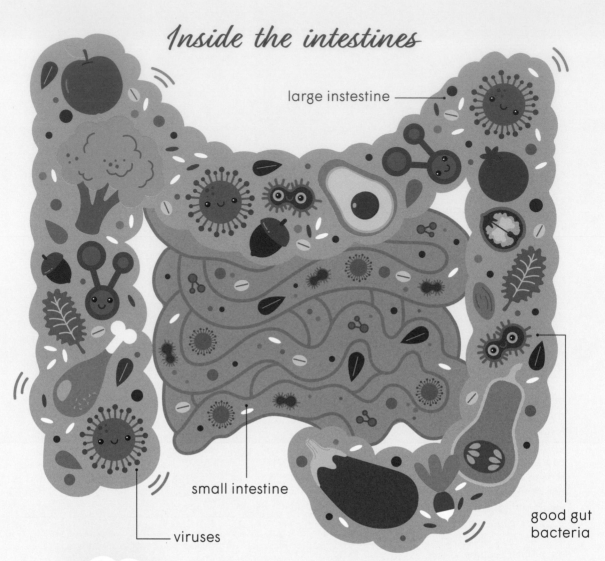

large instestine

small intestine

viruses

good gut bacteria

→ There are as many bacteria cells as there are human cells in your body.
→ These microbes live mainly in the large intestine.
→ They interact with the host (you), taking part in digestion and protection against pathogens.

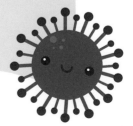

Meet Your Gut
Residents

The human body is more than an organism – it is an ecosystem. It hosts trillions of microorganisms. You contain as many microbes as human cells! Some of these bugs are on your skin, others are in your lungs, but most of them are in your gut – more specifically in the large intestine. And you live in total harmony with them. Together with your microbiome, you form, in fact, a superorganism!

1 Who's there?

Viruses, yeasts, fungi, bacteria, even parasites – all kinds of microorganisms make up your microbiota. And there are lots of them: more than 1000 bacterial species! They are mainly located in your large intestine: about 200 g (7 oz) of microorganisms live in there, the equivalent of an avocado. This is what is called the gut microbiota or microbiome. It might not seem like much, but it carries an enormous amount of genetic material: it encodes over 3 million genes, which is considerable if you compare it to the 23,000 genes that make up the human genome. Genetically, you are more microbe than human!

2 A unique fingerprint

No microbiome resembles another. You have your very own gut microbiota in terms of size, diversity and balance of species, a bit like a unique fingerprint. Although it might change through the course of your life – based on your genes, environment, your lifestyle or your health – it has a memory. It always wants to get back to how it was defined in your childhood.

3 It's all about balance

Like any ecosystem, no one microbiome is better than another. What matters is that the microbiome works well with the host:

→ Does it protect you against pathogens?

→ Does it help you make the most of your food?

→ Does it send the right signals to your brain?

→ Does it respond well to your experience of stress and change of mood?

It is a very personal symbiosis!

Each microbiome is an elaborate equilibrium that self-regulates and adapts according to its environment.

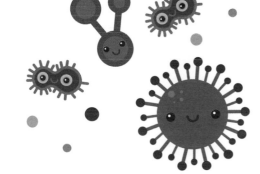

13

The Role of the
Gut Microbiome

Without your gut microbiome, you would get sick all the time, completely vulnerable to parasites and harmful bacteria. This is because your gut microbiome is a key component of your immune system. It also plays an important role in your nutrition. But that's not all – it might even modulate your behaviours and mood.

1 First line of defence

The gut microbiome's main function is defence. First, by competing for space and limited resources in the gut, the microbiota prevents the overgrowth of pathogens that could threaten to invade your body. Certain strains in particular, like Lactobacillus and Bifidobacterium (often found in live yoghurt) are useful because they will inhibit the growth of less desirable bacteria.

Another way your gut microbiome acts as a defence is by interacting with your immune system. It constantly assesses what is travelling through your digestive tract and sends signals to the immune cells advising on:

→ what can safely be let in through your gut barrier

→ what can happily be tolerated in the gut

→ what actually requires a proper immune response, and how strong this response needs to be.

In other words, the gut microbiome trains your immune system to tell friends from foes and then shapes your immune responses.

2 Nutrition

The gut microbiome's other important job is to extract and synthesise more interesting nutrients from the food you eat. By breaking down dietary fibre (a carbohydrate found in plants that we humans can't digest) your bacteria produce essential vitamins like vitamin K and folate, which can then be absorbed. It also facilitates the absorption of minerals such as magnesium, iron and calcium. And finally, it produces some mighty compounds called short-chain fatty acids. When released in the gut, these:

→ strengthen the gut barrier by nourishing the mucous layer of the gut wall – a process that is suspected to reduce the risk of colorectal cancer

→ get absorbed, sending signals to the brain, thus regulating hunger long after your meal.

3 Mood & behaviours

Did you know that your gut bacteria produce neurotransmitters like dopamine and serotonin? In fact, 95 per cent of serotonin – sometimes called the 'happiness hormone' – is secreted in the gut. Serotonin in the gut plays an important role in gut motility (i.e. the speed at which foods travel through the gut) but it also targets the area in the brain involved in mood regulation and cognition. For example, it might affect your experience of stress, your social interactions, your memory and concentration. This is referred to as the gut-brain axis (page 18).

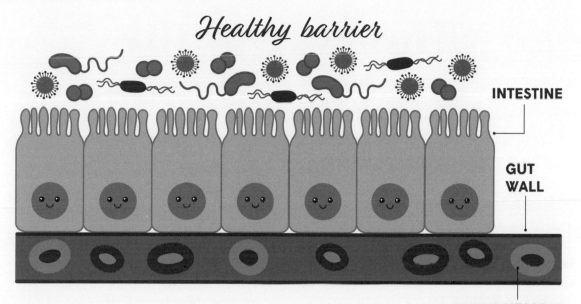

Healthy barrier

INTESTINE

GUT WALL

BLOOD VESSELS

Inflamed leaky barrier

INTESTINE

GUT WALL

BLOOD VESSELS

A healthy gut microbiota creates a thick layer that protects the gut wall – this tight gut barrier prevents pathogens from entering the body, only letting in useful nutrients. But when the gut microbiota is not in great shape, the gut barrier may get disrupted and become more permeable – some microbes might get through and pass into the bloodstream.

A GOOD GUT MICROBIOTA:
- prevents the overgrowth of undesirable microbes
- strengthens the gut barrier
- trains the immune system.

What is a Healthy
Gut Microbiota?

There isn't one ideal microbiome. They come in all kinds, and what is healthy for you might not be right for someone else. But a few characteristics such as stability, size and diversity appear to be key.

1 Stability

Microbes interact with each other, creating a fine balance. Certain strains are particularly beneficial, for example, Bifidobacterium or Lactobacillus found in live yoghurt; while others are potentially dangerous (Clostridium difficile, E. coli). But it would be over-simplistic to say that there are 'bad' bacteria that need to be eliminated. Imagine a sea where there were only plankton and no sharks – it wouldn't work! What is crucial here is stability and equilibrium. Like any ecosystem, all the organisms work together to keep the microbiota stable and optimal for the host – you!

2 Size matters

The bigger the microbiota, the less space there is for harmful microbes to take over and cause damage. A large microbiota seems to improve the whole stability of the ecosystem – the more the merrier!

3 Diversity

A wide range of microbes makes your gut microbiome more capable and resilient. This is because it means a greater diversity in skills: all these microbes produce different metabolites that work for you, doing all kinds of different things. A bit like an organisation, we need all kinds of workers who can be deployed to fight, protect, investigate and strategise. In this community too, diversity is a strength!

4 Shaping your microbiome

Your microbiome is shaped by many factors. Some are out of your control – your genes, your age, the way you were born, whether you were bottle or breastfed, infections you had in the past. But some lifestyle factors may be more within your power: living with pets, spending time in nature, sleeping well and exercising regularly are all beneficial. And obviously, what you eat has a direct and powerful effect on the size, diversity and stability of your microbiome. That's where this book can come in handy!

WHAT ARE METABOLITES?

Small molecules produced from the breakdown – the metabolism – of food or drugs. Metabolites can be nutrients, vitamins, fatty acids, phenols, etc. The digestive system as well as the microbes in the gut produce metabolites, which can then be absorbed by the body or act as signals to other organs.

Healthy gut microbiome

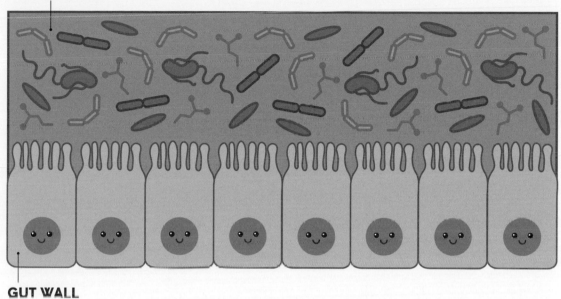

INSIDE THE GUT

GUT WALL

Not so healthy gut microbiome

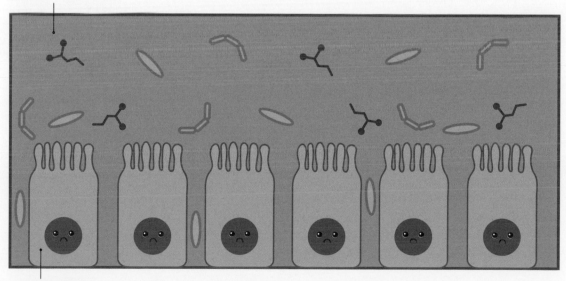

INSIDE THE GUT

GUT WALL

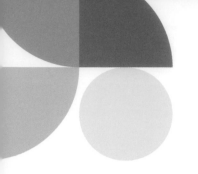

The Gut-brain
Axis

The gut and brain are constantly interacting with each other. The two-way communication influences both your physical and mental well-being, and in your gut, the microbiome plays a key role.

1 A two-way communication

You have probably experienced how emotions have affected your gut in the past: getting butterflies in the stomach when in love; needing to rush to the toilet when feeling stressed. That is the brain 'talking' to the gut. But communication goes the other way too. You know that 'gut feeling'? The gut microbiota constantly sends signals to tell the brain to 'feel' a certain way.

2 Promising lab work

Studies on rodents have consistently shown that the gut microbiome's activity can influence the brain. When studying germ-free mice (i.e. mice without a microbiota), scientists noticed that the animals were behaving strangely compared to normal mice: they were more fearless, less sociable and more aggressive with others. Yet, when bacteria were placed into their gut (using a technique called faecal microbiome transplant), the mice's behaviour would become 'normal'. In other words, the presence of gut microbiota changed their behaviour. Such findings are very interesting … but mainly for rodents!

3 And for humans?

Obviously, we can't study germ-free humans! But scientists have carried out promising experiments. For example, the SMILES trial has shown that giving a diet rich in dietary fibre (the carbohydrates that we can't digest but that our gut microbiota thrives on) to people suffering from depression, in addition to their existing treatments, led to significant alleviation of their depression and anxiety symptoms. Food is powerful stuff!

4 Other connections

And there is more evidence that gut and mood are linked: unhealthy diets (high in processed foods and low in plant-based foods) are associated with a higher risk of developing depression or anxiety. It's the same story with disorders such as dementia.

But let's be cautious in drawing conclusions. If research links diet and gut microbiome to various activities in the brain, it doesn't mean that diet can cure Alzheimer's or even keep depression at bay – the brain is a complex thing, and so many factors are at play.

These findings suggest that taking care of your gut microbiome is one tool you have to support your mental well-being. Every little bit helps!

How the gut may talk to the brain

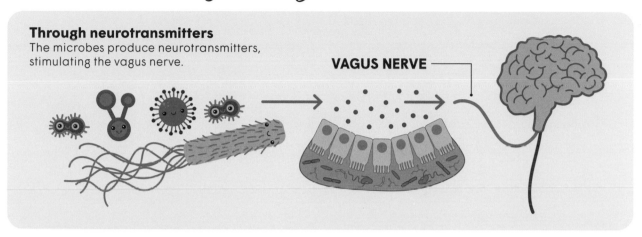

Through neurotransmitters
The microbes produce neurotransmitters, stimulating the vagus nerve.

VAGUS NERVE

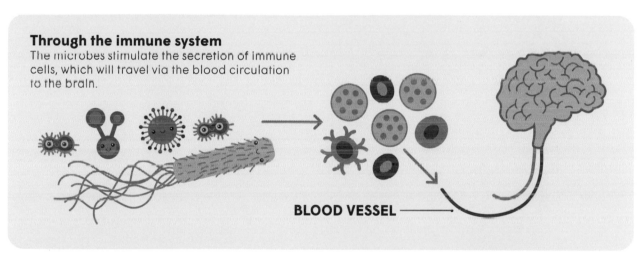

Through the immune system
The microbes stimulate the secretion of immune cells, which will travel via the blood circulation to the brain.

BLOOD VESSEL

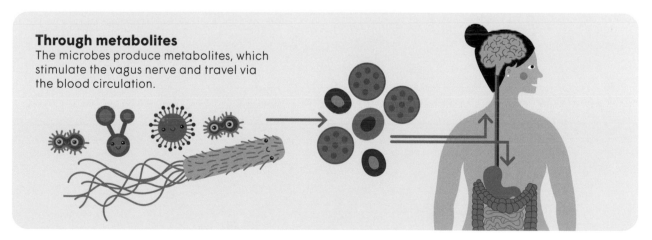

Through metabolites
The microbes produce metabolites, which stimulate the vagus nerve and travel via the blood circulation.

Diseases associated with gut dysbiosis

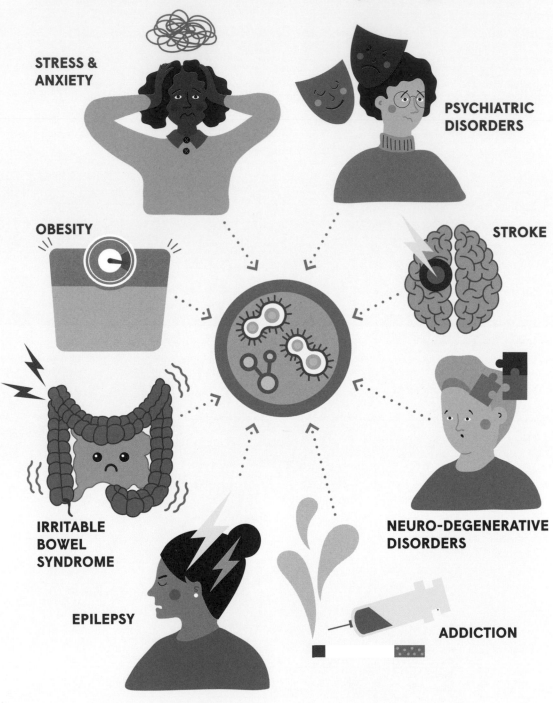

STRESS & ANXIETY

PSYCHIATRIC DISORDERS

OBESITY

STROKE

IRRITABLE BOWEL SYNDROME

NEURO-DEGENERATIVE DISORDERS

EPILEPSY

ADDICTION

Microbiome
& Disease

Depending on whether you are ill or healthy, your microbiome will look different. Changes may be temporary – you and your gut will bounce back quickly, but sometimes the damage can become bedded-in, as is the case with chronic diseases.

❶ A fragile ecosystem

Your microbiome is like any ecosystem: it is dynamic and adaptable. It constantly changes depending on the time of the day, what you eat, what medicines you take, how much you sleep, etc. – much as a forest changes depending on the climate and the season.

❷ When it goes wrong

At times the gut microbiome's equilibrium gets damaged and the microbiome suffers. This is known as 'dysbiosis' and is often associated with physical symptoms (e.g. diarrhoea, rash). The microbiome then tends to become smaller in size, with more inflammatory bacteria. It also lacks diversity, presenting fewer strains of microbes. This happens after you have had a bacterial infection, or when you have taken antibiotics for example. Luckily, dysbiosis is usually temporary. The microbiome has a memory and, if allowed, will slowly return to its initial and natural state of balance.

❸ Long-term damage

But this is not always the case. In fact, a state of microbiome dysbiosis has been implicated in all kinds of non-communicable diseases:

→ allergies and autoimmune diseases, such as asthma, eczema, Coeliac disease, multiple sclerosis, rheumatoid arthritis

→ metabolic diseases, such as obesity, type 1 and 2 diabetes, heart disease

→ neuro-degenerative and cognitive disorders, such as autism, Alzheimer's

→ mood disorders, such as anxiety, depression

→ bowel issues, such as irritable bowel syndrome (IBS), inflammatory bowel disease (IBD), colon cancer

→ addiction

→ epilepsy.

❹ The gut is linked to so many disorders!

What isn't clear yet is the role of the gut microbiota in those diseases. Is it the illness that induces dysbiosis of the microbiome? Or does the dysbiosis facilitate the development of the illness? One thing is sure; by taking care of your gut microbiome, you can support your immune system and strengthen your well-being.

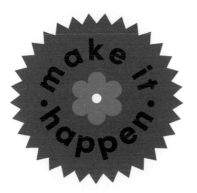

What Shapes our
Gut Microbiota?

The gut microbiota is like a fingerprint – it is unique to an individual, but it evolves through time and changes in response to its environment.

1 First steps of life

The first 1000 days of life – from conception until the end of the second year – are crucial in shaping the gut microbiota and in the baby's immune system development.

→ The first colonisation of the gut happens before birth, in the womb, through the placenta.

→ The second stage occurs at birth where the hospital setting and the mode of delivery matters. The more sterile the environment, the smaller the colonisation. A natural birth is, in that aspect, preferable to a Caesarean section.

→ The third wave of colonisation happens during infancy, through skin-to-skin contact but, above all, through breast milk. That milk acts as a prebiotic (page 32) as it enables existing beneficial bacteria to thrive while tempering the growth of more harmful ones.

→ The final developmental stage in the child's microbiota comes with the gradual introduction of solid foods.

2 The age of stability

By the age of three, the microbiome has reached maturity. Throughout adulthood, it might respond slightly to your environment, your habits and your health but, overall, it will stay fairly stable for many years until you reach 60.

3 Getting old

It is only towards the end of life that it starts to change, losing diversity and richness, and making the host a bit more vulnerable: the immune system gets weaker, levels of inflammation are higher, response to vaccination is reduced. The gut microbiota is ageing at the same time as the body.

4 Nothing is set in stone

Although the main characteristics of your microbiome have been defined in the early stages of your life, there are many things that can change its composition (its size and diversity). Medication, physical activity, diet – all of these may promote the development of some bacteria over others and slightly change the ecosystem's equilibrium for the better … or for the worse!

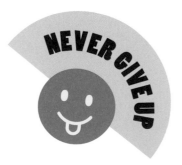

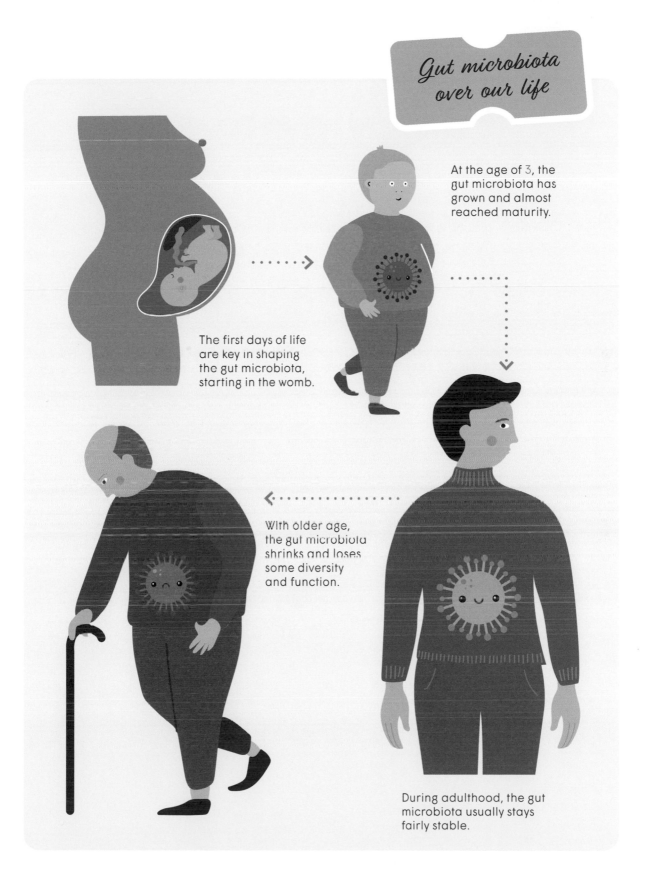

Gut microbiota
over our life

At the age of 3, the gut microbiota has grown and almost reached maturity.

The first days of life are key in shaping the gut microbiota, starting in the womb.

With older age, the gut microbiota shrinks and loses some diversity and function.

During adulthood, the gut microbiota usually stays fairly stable.

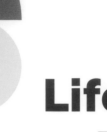

Lifestyle Habits
That Count

Your gut microbiota has a memory of what it likes to be – so it can be really difficult to completely transform it. But external factors can knock it back or make it thrive, which means that by paying attention to what is within your control, you can tweak it to work better for you.

Like any living organism, the gut microbiome is very sensitive to its surrounding conditions. Here are a few factors that may affect it:

1 Medications

These may knock out some of the microorganisms in the gut, leaving space for more harmful species to take over. This is why it might be a good idea to take a probiotic alongside a course of antibiotics, for example.

2 Smoking

This doesn't only harm your lungs, it also harms your gut microbiome! It affects the gut permeability (making the normally tight barrier of the gut wall a bit looser) and increases inflammation. Luckily, this can be reversed when you stop smoking.

3 Chronic stress

Rather than occasional stress, chronic stress can disrupt the balance of the microbiome, leaving the gut more vulnerable and irritable. Stress management activities like yoga, meditation, breathing and hypnotherapy can do wonders to re-establish the gut balance.

4 Poor sleep

Whether it is due to jet lag, sleep deprivation or shift work, poor sleep will hurt your microbiota, because, like any of your body organs, it follows a wake–sleep rhythm in sync with the day–night cycle. Taking care of your sleep hygiene to ensure 7–9 hours' sleep, uninterrupted and at night-time, will be very much appreciated by your gut residents!

5 Physical activity

This is wonderful at stimulating the growth of good bacteria. So, keep your body moving and explore ways to get that heart pumping, no matter what your age. Find a sport or activity that you like and make sure it is part of your daily/weekly routine, with some regular periods of rest to allow your body to recover … and your microbiome.

6 Nature & pets

Because they expose you to different microorganisms, spending time in nature or with your pets will increase the diversity of your gut microbiota. That is why it is so important to get outside, connect with nature and give that pup a hug.

7 Diet

Finally, diet is a wonderful and powerful tool to tweak and steer the shape of your gut microbiome: what you choose to eat can not only provide the nutrients needed by the microorganisms to thrive, but it can also bring new and more beneficial bacteria to your gut.

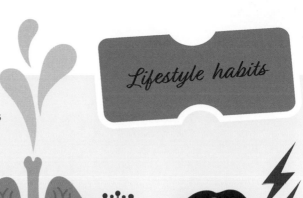

Smoking stimulates gut inflammation and damages the lining of your bowels.

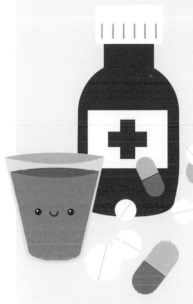

Medication such as antibiotics can wipe out your gut microbiota.

Chronic stress disrupts the balance of your gut microbiota.

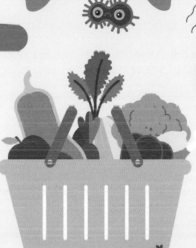

Diet is one tool you have to help shape your gut microbiome.

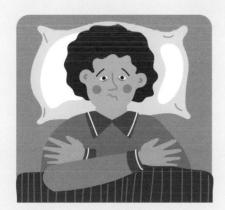

Lack of sleep can negatively affect the microbiome equilibrium.

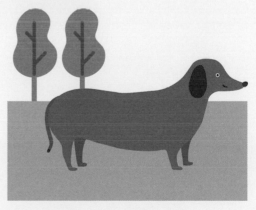

Nature gives a diversity boost to the range of microbes in your gut.

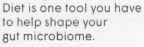

Foods for a Thriving
Gut Microbiota

By following a few simple principles and tweaking your diet, you can do wonders for your gut and its residents. A great way to start is by adding more plants to your plate.

1 Plants, more plants

Let's be clear: there's no need to go vegan, at least as far as gut health is concerned, but it's worth focusing on bringing more plants to your plate. This is because the microorganisms that live in your gut LOVE them. In particular, they love dietary fibre. Fibre is a type of carbohydrate found in plants, but unlike other carbs (sugar, starch) your body is unable to break it down – you just don't have the right enzyme to digest and extract energy from it. The good news though: your gut microbiota can, and they do! They feast on fibre, fuelling their growth in numbers.

2 Even more plants

It is not only fibre that is good in plants, there are also phytochemicals ('phyto' meaning from plants) with antioxidative properties. These polyphenols stimulate the growth of the right kind of microorganisms and also strengthen the gut barrier.

3 Some fermented foods

If dietary fibre is considered the 'fertiliser' for gut microorganisms, fermented foods are the 'seeds'. Fermented foods such as yoghurt and sauerkraut are full of live bacteria. By eating these foods some bacteria will reach your colon and settle there, adding more volume and diversity to your gut microbiota.

4 A bit of interesting fat

Omega-3, a type of polyunsaturated fat, is particularly good because it increases the quantity of beneficial bacteria known for their ability to produce short-chain fatty acids and positively stimulate the gut-brain axis. Omega-3 fat can be found in oily fish (e.g. salmon, mackerel, sardines, tuna, trout), as well as in plant-based foods like walnuts, linseeds (flax seeds) and chia seeds. Finally, don't forget olive oil. This monounsaturated fat also does wonders for your gut.

5 Stay hydrated

It is not only food that keeps the gut microbiota in good shape, water is also important, lowering the numbers of potentially harmful bacteria and creating the perfect conditions for your ecosystem to thrive.

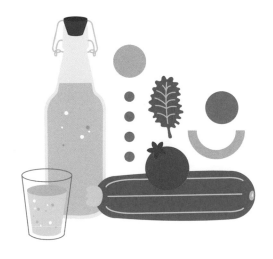

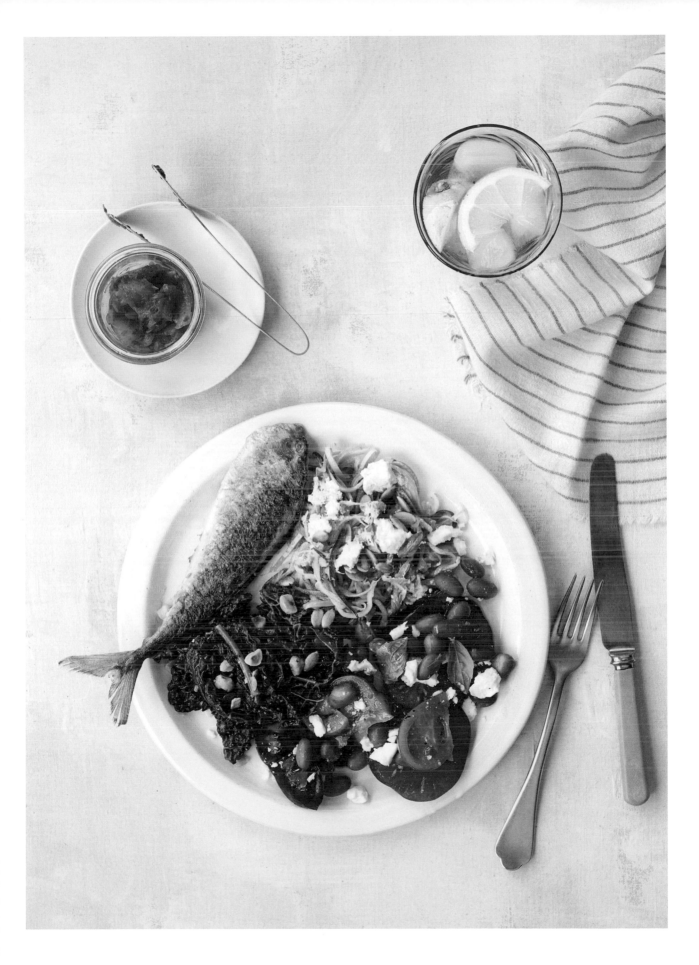

Checklist for daily minimal target (30 g dietary fibre):

Fibre-rich food	Quantities	Fibre content
2 portions of fruit	1 apple	4.4 g
	2 kiwi fruits	5 g
5 portions of vegetables	½ eggplant/aubergine (with skin)	7 g
	spinach leaves	2 g
	1 tomato	1.5 g
	3 broccoli florets	2.5 g
	½ sweet potato (with skin)	3 g
3 portions of wholegrains	1 bowl of porridge	4 g
	1 serving of brown rice	3.5 g
	1 slice of multigrain bread	3 g
2 portions of nuts, seeds or legumes	1 handful of almonds	3.5 g
	1 serving of lentils	6.5 g

→ Portions of **fruit** or **vegetable**: size of a **fist**

→ Portions of **wholegrains**: size of a **fist**

→ Portions of **nuts**: a **small handful**

→ Portions of **seeds**: **1 tablespoon**

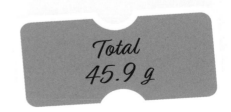

Total
45.9 g

The Benefits of
Dietary Fibre

Fibre, the non-digestible carbohydrate found in plants, is key to a happy gut. But there isn't just one kind of fibre – there are over 100. Different fibres have very different health effects and functions.

1 Poop regulation

Soluble fibre dissolves slowly in the gut creating a thick, jelly-like texture. This slows down the digestion and will help with creating the perfect poop: not too runny, not too hard. It is also associated with lower levels of cholesterol and better blood glucose levels. It is found in oats, barley, beans, lentils, peas and apples.

Insoluble fibre adds bulk to the stool, speeding up the passing of food through the gut. It gets things moving! It is found in the skin of fruit and vegetables, in wholegrains, seeds and nuts.

2 Fascinating fermentation

Some fibres, such as resistant starch, are highly fermentable, which means that they get broken down by the gut microbiota – it is their fuel. Not only do such fibres enable the microbes to thrive but, through the process of fermentation, they produce something wonderful: short-chain fatty acids. These metabolites are the ingredient for good health beyond the gut: they modulate the immune function, influence hormone secretion and stimulate the nervous system.

Fermentable fibre is found in potatoes, green bananas, wholegrains, pulses, legumes, cashew nuts and oats.

3 The more the better – but not any old how

The current recommendation is to aim for at least 30 g of fibre per day, yet currently the average adult in Europe gets only 15–20 g daily. There is clearly room for improvement! Better health results have been associated with a much higher amount of dietary fibre (around 50 g a day).

However, there are two precautions when increasing the amount of fibre in your diet:

→ First, fibre should be added gradually to allow the gut to adjust to these changes. Otherwise, the sudden feast in the large intestine might come with some discomfort such as bloating and gas.

→ Second, since some fibre will draw a lot of water into the gut, it is important to increase your hydration to avoid cramps.

DID YOU KNOW?

Plant skin is a great source of fibre, so don't peel everything. Banana skin might not be to everyone's taste, but do keep the skin on apples, cucumbers, eggplant (aubergines) and sweet potatoes.

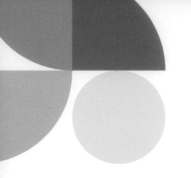

Diversity First
& Foremost

Different types of fibre feed different microorganisms. This means that a diet with a broad range of plants will lead to greater diversity of microbes in the gut. And the greater the gut microbiota diversity, the better the gut health. So, why not try something new?

1 The 30-plant challenge

Research from the American Gut Microbiome project showed that people who ate more than 30 different plant-based foods per week had a much more diverse gut microbiota compared to those who ate less than 10 plants per week. So, are you ready for the 30-plant challenge? It is much easier than it sounds. Think of fruit, vegetables, wholegrains, nuts, seeds, pulses, herbs and spices. It all counts!

2 Here are some ideas: Easy add-ons

Having cereal for breakfast? Top it with a few berries and nuts.

Snacking on an apple? Chop it and dip it into the nut butter of your choice.

Eating a sandwich for lunch? Tuck in a few leaves of rocket (arugula).

Serving soup for dinner? Scatter some seeds and herbs on top.

Planning to roast some vegetables? Season them with various spices (cumin, smoked paprika, ground turmeric).

Making a bolognese for the family? Halve the amount of meat and add some lentils or beans instead. Add some sweet potato and zucchini (courgette) for good measure.

3 Easy swaps

Always eating the same white bread? Swap for wholegrain and vary the grain: how about trying rye or spelt?

Regularly snacking on cashew nuts? Swap for almonds or walnuts.

Broccoli is your go-to vegetable? Try Romanesco broccoli or cauliflower.

Eating a lot of rice? Try brown, wild, black or red rice.

Making chicken goujon? Swap the breadcrumbs for milled oats or crushed cereal.

Check out the recipes in this book (pages 64–150). They are full of fibre-packed foods, using different grains, a wide variety of nuts and seeds and lots of herb toppings so you should easily eat 30 different plants a week, and more!

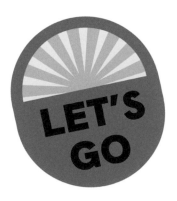

LET'S GO

Try the 30-plant challenge

VEGETABLES

Artichokes
Asparagus
Beetroot (beets)
Bell peppers (capsicums)
Brussels sprouts
Broccoli
Butternut squash
Carrots
Cauliflower
Eggplant
(aubergines)
French shallots
Garlic
Green beans
Leeks
Olives
Parsnips
Pointed cabbage
Pumpkin (winter squash)
Red onions
Russian kale
Spinach
Spring greens
Swede (rutabaga)
Sweet potatoes
Sweetcorn
Tomatoes
Turnips
Yellow zucchini (courgettes)

FRUIT

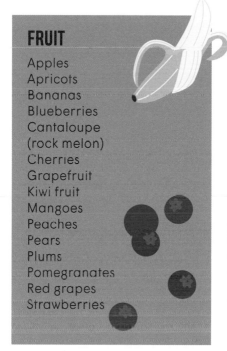

Apples
Apricots
Bananas
Blueberries
Cantaloupe
(rock melon)
Cherries
Grapefruit
Kiwi fruit
Mangoes
Peaches
Pears
Plums
Pomegranates
Red grapes
Strawberries

WHOLEGRAINS

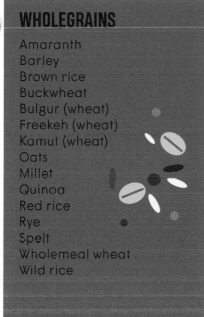

Amaranth
Barley
Brown rice
Buckwheat
Bulgur (wheat)
Freekeh (wheat)
Kamut (wheat)
Oats
Millet
Quinoa
Red rice
Rye
Spelt
Wholemeal wheat
Wild rice

LEGUMES

Beluga lentils
Black beans
Black-eyed peas
Borlotti (cranberry) beans
Cannellini beans
Chickpeas (garbanzo
beans)
Kidney beans
Lupin beans
Mung beans
Peanuts
Pinto beans
Puy lentils
Red lentils
Soy beans
Split peas

HERBS & SPICES

Basil
Chives
Coriander (cilantro)
Dill
Lemongrass
Mint
Oregano
Parsley
Rosemary
Tarragon
Thyme
Black pepper
Cardamom
Chilli
Cinnamon
Coriander seed
Cumin
Ginger
Mustard
Nutmeg
Smoked paprika
Turmeric

NUTS & SEEDS

Almonds
Brazil nuts
Cashews
Chia seeds
Hazelnuts
Linseeds (flax seeds)
Macadamias
Pistachios
Pumpkin seeds
Sesame seeds
Sunflower seeds
Walnuts

Prebiotics,
food for our gut microbes

Although all types of dietary fibre are great for your gut, make sure you specifically include the best ones – the ones that good bacteria (i.e. the ones known to have health benefits) love to feed on. These are called prebiotics (not to be confused with probiotics – more on those later).

1 Some mighty fibres

All prebiotics are fibres, but not all dietary fibres are prebiotics. To be a prebiotic, the fibre needs to be fermentable – in other words it needs to be edible by the gut microbes. Secondly, it needs to be proven to modify, for the better, the composition and function of the gut microbiota. Currently, the main prebiotics that have been identified are inulin, oligofructose (OF), galacto-oligosaccharides (GOS) and fructo-oligosaccharides (FOS). You might see these names mentioned on gut-friendly foods' labels.

2 Health benefits

Prebiotics are an easy way to support our health. They are thought to help with digestion, appetite regulation, blood glucose levels, immune function and mineral absorption. They may also help with mood regulation, cognitive functions (memory and learning) and stress management. Interestingly, a lot of prebiotics are present in breast milk and play a key role in supporting a newborn's health, right from the beginning.

3 Prebiotic-rich foods

Prebiotics can be found in a wide range of fruit, vegetables, grains, nuts and legumes. Here are some great sources:

→ **Vegetables:** asparagus, chicory root, Jerusalem artichokes, leeks, onions, garlic

→ **Fruit:** dried figs, dried mango, apricots, green bananas, prunes, nectarines

→ **Grains:** oats, barley, rye, spelt

→ **Nuts:** almonds, cashew nuts, pistachios, hazelnuts

→ **Legumes:** black beans, chickpeas (garbanzo beans), butter beans (lima beans).

4 Go slow

Like any fibre, it is important to introduce prebiotics progressively in the diet to avoid discomfort such as gas or bloating. The body – and the gut microbiota – need a bit of time to adapt to this change in diet.

5 How about a pill?

You might have seen prebiotics offered as food supplements, but it is currently not very clear how helpful they are. The best strategy by far is to focus on prebiotic-rich foods, as this will certainly be celebrated in your gut.

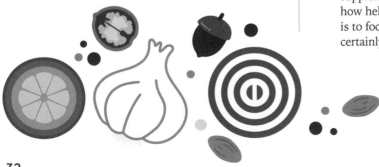

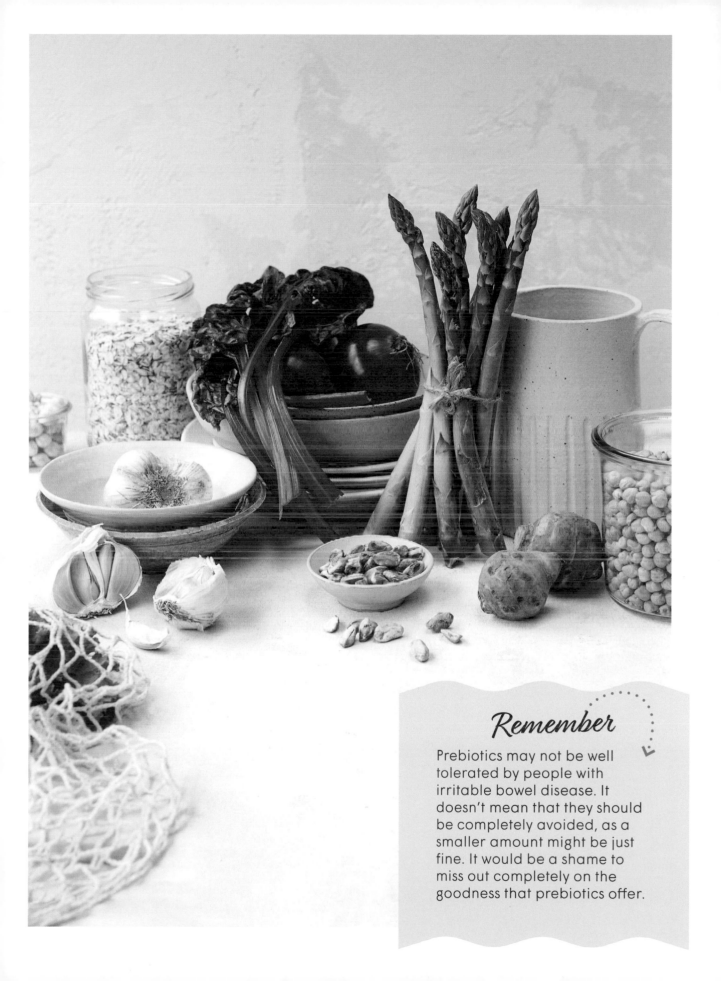

Remember

Prebiotics may not be well tolerated by people with irritable bowel disease. It doesn't mean that they should be completely avoided, as a smaller amount might be just fine. It would be a shame to miss out completely on the goodness that prebiotics offer.

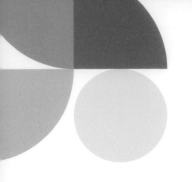

The Power
of Colours

Besides dietary fibre, there is another family of components from plant food that's worth paying attention to: polyphenols. These bio-active phytochemicals are often praised for their antioxidant properties. They also appear to modulate the activity of our gut microbiota for the better.

1 Eat the rainbow

Resveratrol from red wine and raspberries, curcuma from turmeric, flavanols from cocoa and tea, tannins from tea and coffee, anthocyanins from berries and red cabbage … there are hundreds of polyphenols in nature, often linked to the tastes, aromas and colours of the plants. Hence, the importance of eating foods of all different colours. They are widely found in fruit, vegetables, legumes, herbs, seeds and spices.

2 Health benefits

Scientists think that these polyphenols may have powerful protective effects against diseases such as diabetes, obesity, neurodegenerative disorders, cardiovascular diseases and even certain cancers. But how could they work?

3 The role of the gut microbiome

Only a small amount of polyphenols is absorbed during digestion in the small intestine. The bulk of them gets broken down by the gut microbiota in the colon, a process which produces lots of active metabolites (page 16). It is these metabolites that will have anti-inflammatory, anti-allergenic and anticarcinogenic effects, so, bring colours to your plate!

4 Shaping the microbiota too

The presence of these polyphenols will also influence the composition of your gut microbiota: they stimulate the growth of the beneficial microbes while keeping under control the proliferation of the more harmful ones. By having lots of polyphenol-rich food in your diet, you really strengthen the balance, size and stability of your gut microbiome.

TIP

Light stimulates the production of polyphenols so they are often concentrated in the outer layer, such as the skin and leaves. This is another good reason not to peel fruit and vegetables, and to sprinkle your plate with lots of fresh herbs.

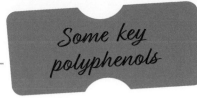
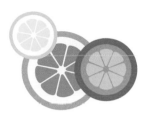

Flavanones
These may help with inflammation in the body and help protect it against toxins. They are found in lemons, grapefruits and oranges.

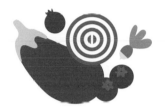

Anthocyanins
These are usually found in the outer skin of fruit and vegetables including pomegranates, red cabbage, red onions, blueberries, radishes and eggplants (aubergines).

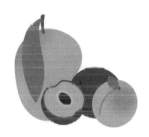

Isoflavones
These are also known as phytoestrogens (they are similar in structure to oestrogen) and are found in soy beans, apricots, mangoes, plums and sesame seeds.

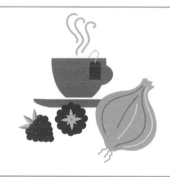

Phenolic acids
These may have anti-inflammatory properties and are found in a wide range of plant-based foods including strawberries, blackberries, tea, onions and tomatoes.

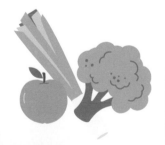

Flavanols
These have antioxidant properties and may help lower blood pressure and can manage symptoms of cardiovascular disease. They are found in broccoli, curly kale, leeks, apples and green tea.

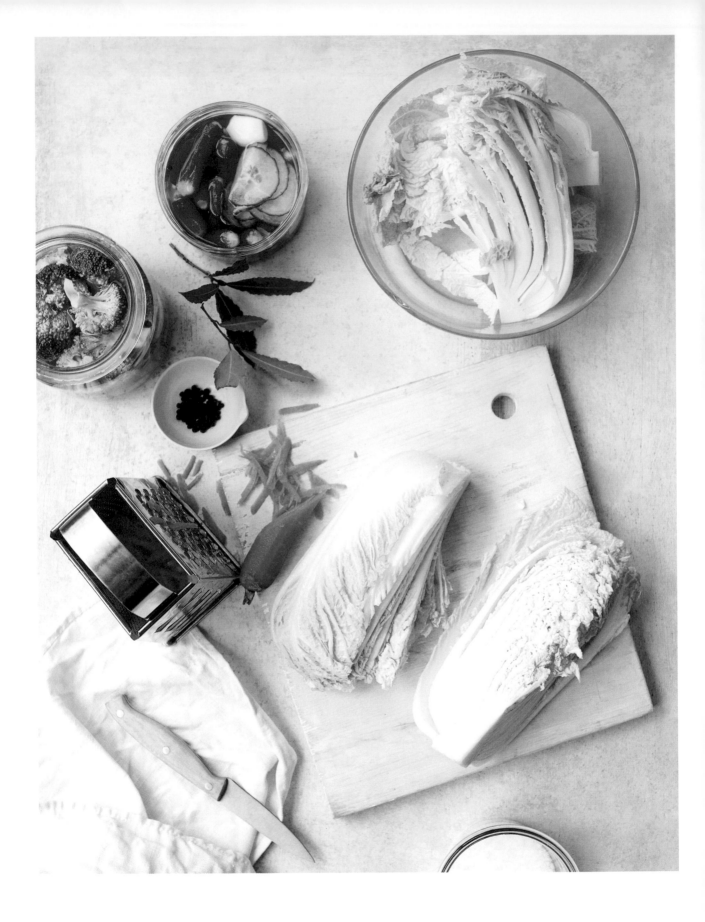

Fermented
Foods

Fermentation has been around for thousands of years as a technique to preserve food and increase its shelf life. But wait, there's much more to it!

❶ The fermentation process

The principle of lacto-fermentation is simple: by stimulating the growth of harmless yeast or bacteria in an airtight container it inhibits the proliferation of pathogens and prevents the food from spoiling. What happens in the sauerkraut jar is very much like what happens in your gut. The bacteria feed on the carbohydrates (fibre for kimchi, milk for yoghurt) and multiply, breaking down food molecules and producing by-products like gas and bio-active compounds such as lactic acid and vitamins.

❷ Delicious & highly digestible

This transformation improves the texture and the taste of the food, giving a sour, tangy and sometimes even fizzy flavour. It also changes the molecular structure of the food. For example, the lactose molecules in yoghurt (or in fermented cheese) are broken down by the bacteria making it much more digestible for people with lactose intolerance. It is the same with sourdough bread: because of its fermentation, it is often much better tolerated by wheat-sensitive people. It also enhances the nutrition value of the food through the synthesis of vitamins and other biologically active molecules.

❸ Sowing the seeds

Fermented foods, as long as they haven't been cooked or pasteurised, are a great source of live microorganisms. By eating live microbes – a bit like sowing seeds in a garden – some will flourish in your gut, adding volume and diversity to your existing gut microbiota.

❹ What to eat

To give your gut microbiota a boost, choose foods that have retained their live microbes (check for 'live culture' on the label):

→ yoghurt, kefir, cheese
→ sauerkraut, kimchi and other lacto-fermented (pickled) vegetables
→ drinks, such as kombucha, some beers
→ fermented soy products, such as miso, natto, tempeh.

Fermented foods that are cooked or pasteurised won't have any live microorganisms any more but will have retained their higher digestibility:

→ sourdough bread
→ wine, most beers
→ soy sauce
→ coffee and chocolate beans.

Probiotics,
your gut's good guys

Some bacteria turn out to be particularly helpful, healthwise, and can be found in some fermented foods or in food supplements. Are you ready to give them a go?

1 Probiotic-containing foods

A lot of fermented foods such as kefir, live yoghurt and kimchi will contain amounts of these beneficial live microorganisms – and yet, they may not be called probiotics. This is because products need to meet three rigorous criteria:

→ The microbes need to be alive.

→ The strains need to have documented health benefits.

→ They must be present in large amounts.

So, if the kefir from the supermarket doesn't say 'probiotic', this doesn't mean that it won't have any health benefit – rather, the manufacturer wasn't able to guarantee that the three criteria were met. They are producing food, after all, not medicine.

2 Probiotics as supplements

You can also find probiotics as food supplements. These can certainly be useful, especially when:

→ you take them alongside a course of antibiotics

→ you have gut issues such as irritable bowel syndrome, diarrhoea, or you are at risk of inflammatory bowel disease (Crohn's disease, ulcerative colitis)

→ you are healthy but want to prevent some illnesses.

Probiotics are considered safe to use by adults but do check with a healthcare professional if you are pregnant, have a compromised immune system, or would like to use them for a child.

3 Be strategic

Here are a few things to keep in mind:

→ Different strains will have different health benefits, so be specific when choosing your probiotic and ask for help from a healthcare professional.

→ **Not all probiotics will have been clinically tested**: the right strains might be present in large amounts, but will they arrive in sufficient numbers in the gut? Choose a reliable brand and check if it has been properly tested.

→ Not everyone will get benefits from the same probiotic – the microbiome is still a big, unknown field, and it is hard to know what will have an effect or not.

DEFINITION

Probiotic (not to be confused with 'prebiotic', page 32) is the name given to any live microorganism that, when taken in adequate amounts, has been shown to provide health benefits. They may help with diarrhoea, constipation or bloating; with irritable bowel symptoms and managing cholesterol levels.

7 benefits of good gut bacteria

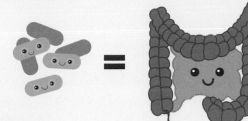

Gut barrier
Protects and strengthens the gut wall, which may prevent inflammation and some types of cancers.

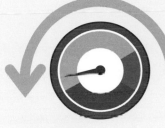

pH levels
Reduces slightly the pH levels in the colon and prevents infections.

Harmful invaders
Can prevent bad bacteria invading the body through the gut.

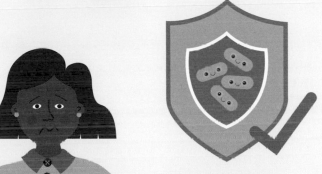

immune function
Trains the immune system on how to respond to pathogens.

Diarrhoea
May help to relieve the occurrence and duration of diarrhoea caused by illness or antibiotics.

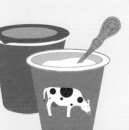

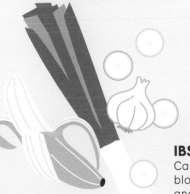

Nutrition
Helps with extracting more nutrients from the food you have eaten.

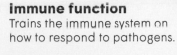

IBS symptoms
Can help to reduce bloating, abdominal pain and improve stool shape in people with IBS.

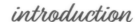

Foods to
Watch Out For

A lot of foods will nourish your gut microbiota and encourage good bacteria to thrive, but are there foods that can knock it back? Absolutely, and not necessarily the ones you might think though.

❶ Alcohol – not great for your gut health

Excess alcohol messes up the whole gut: it damages digestion and unsettles the whole ecosystem by stimulating the growth of some bacteria while reducing others. The imbalance may increase the permeability of the gut and promote inflammation. Luckily, these changes are usually quickly reversed once alcohol has been cleared from the system.

❷ Salt – probably not helpful either

A diet high in salt is suspected to reduce the numbers of good bacteria such as Lactobacilli, while low-salt diets show higher levels of these health-promoting short-chain fatty acids produced by the gut microbiota. Being careful with salt is probably a good idea.

❸ White sugar – probably OK

There are a lot of misconceptions about white sugar. It is true that too much sugar can mess up your blood glucose levels and damage your teeth, so it should be eaten in moderation, but, when eaten in small amounts, sugar has very little impact on your gut and its inhabitants. This is because sugar gets absorbed quite early during digestion (have you ever noticed the almost instant boost of energy that a handful of jelly beans gives you?). By the time food reaches the large intestine where the bulk of the gut microbiota is, not much sugar is left, if any. White sugar in reasonable amounts is very unlikely to be the real cause of gut disorders.

❹ Artificial sweeteners – maybe OK, maybe not

Sucralose, aspartame, saccharin – these artificial sweeteners are popular because they sweeten without adding extra calories to a dish, since they simply can't be absorbed by humans. This means that, unlike table sugar, they do end up in the large intestine. Several studies in animals have shown that they damaged their gut microbiota, but human studies are less clear-cut. It seems as if artificial sweeteners might be problematic for some, while well tolerated by others.

❺ Limitation rather than avoidance

Some foods might have a negative impact on the gut microbiota, but this doesn't mean they should be avoided completely. In nutrition, balance is crucial and excluding food should always be considered carefully. This is because there is more than just gut health to take into account. Mental health, growth and repair, muscle performance, cardiovascular health, nervous system function, etc. – the body is a complex system. It needs all kinds of nutrients to function optimally. So rather than thinking in terms of good or bad food, you would be better off considering your overall diet and how it covers all your body's needs.

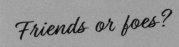

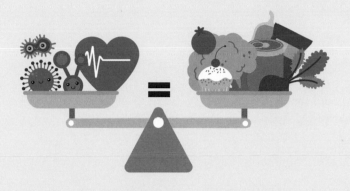

Healthy diet
balanced

Eating very little sugar
positive

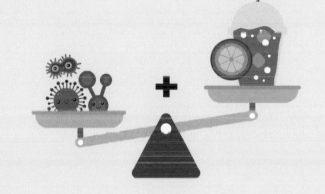

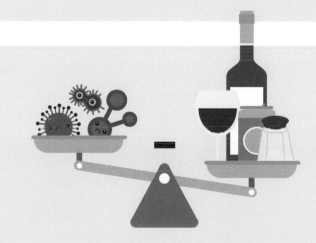

Drinking alcohol
negative

The Western Diet:
Not So Gut Friendly

Do you eat mainly processed foods, or do you prefer cooking from scratch? Hopefully it is the latter. The Western diet that emerged in the 1970s, with the rise of fast foods and ready-meals, is sadly, not great news for our gut-dwellers.

People who eat a classic Western diet have a rather poor gut microbiota:

→ fewer microbes in the large intestine

→ a smaller range of microorganisms

→ fewer good bacteria.

Unsurprisingly, it comes with health issues: high levels of inflammation, cognitive and mood disorders, higher insulin resistance, obesity.

1 Hallmarks of a Western diet

The typical characteristics of a Western diet are:

→ high in ultra-processed foods: soft drinks, hotdogs, savoury snacks, confectionery, breakfast cereals

→ high in saturated fat: bacon, sausage rolls, cookies, pastries

→ high in animal-based foods: meat, charcuterie, dairy products

→ high in refined sugar: soft drinks, juices, sweetened yoghurt, breakfast cereals, cookies, chocolate bars

→ low in fruit and vegetables

→ low in pulses, nuts and seeds

→ low in wholegrains.

2 Starving microbes

The issue with the Western diet is that, because most of the carbohydrates are fast-released sugars and it contains minimal fibre, it provides very little food for your good gut bacteria to thrive.

On the other hand, this diet is high in fat and meat. Part of these foods will make their way into the large intestine, ready to feed the microbiota. But unfortunately, they won't be turned into those beneficial metabolites that are short-chain fatty acids like dietary fibre would. Meat and fat also stimulate the growth of more harmful bacteria, creating an environment prone to inflammation.

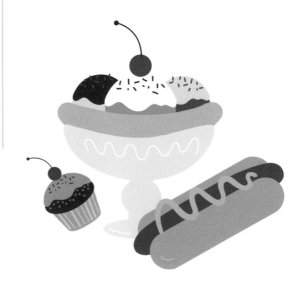

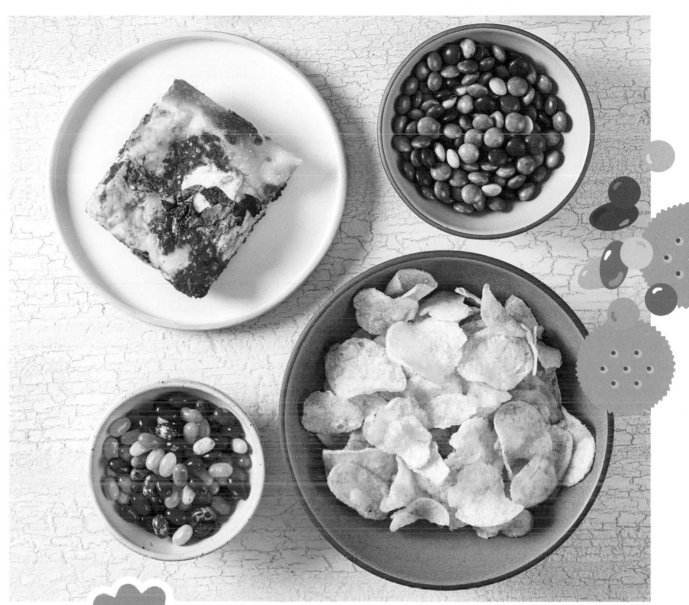

Ultra-processed foods

These are a type of foods that are created using substances extracted from other foods (e.g. fats, sugar, starch, proteins), with added ingredients to improve their palatability (e.g. flavour enhancers), their appearance (e.g. food colourings) and/or their shelf life (e.g. preservatives). In other words, these are foods that have lots of unfamiliar ingredients listed at the back of the packets and that you would struggle to cook from scratch in your kitchen.

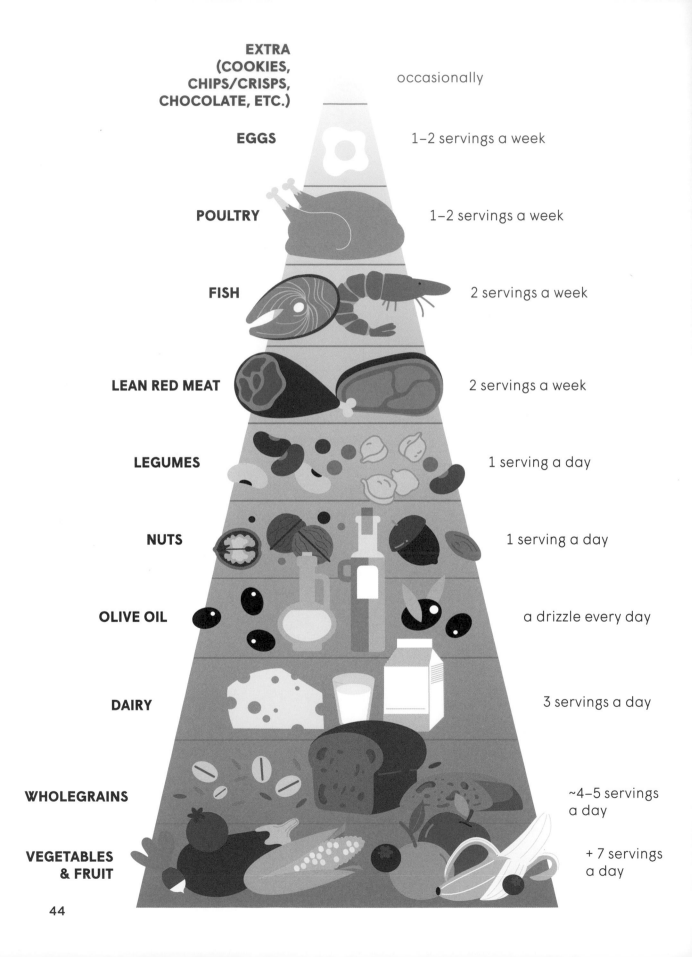

EXTRA (COOKIES, CHIPS/CRISPS, CHOCOLATE, ETC.) — occasionally

EGGS — 1–2 servings a week

POULTRY — 1–2 servings a week

FISH — 2 servings a week

LEAN RED MEAT — 2 servings a week

LEGUMES — 1 serving a day

NUTS — 1 serving a day

OLIVE OIL — a drizzle every day

DAIRY — 3 servings a day

WHOLEGRAINS — ~4–5 servings a day

VEGETABLES & FRUIT — + 7 servings a day

Gut-friendly
Diets

Diets rich in plants, such as the Mediterranean diet or a vegetarian diet, are great for the gut. Just make sure that they have all the nutrients you need to thrive.

1 The Mediterranean diet

The Mediterranean diet, rich in all kinds of plant-based foods, has been studied extensively, showing great results on the gut microbiome: a larger volume of microbes in the gut, a broader range of strains and specifically lots of the good ones. But a good diet is more than just a list of foods. Variety and portions matter too.

2 Hallmarks of the Mediterranean diet

Here is what a gut-friendly Mediterranean diet looks like:

→ high in plant-based foods: a wide range of fruit, vegetables, lentils, beans, peas, nuts, seeds and cereals

→ high in unsaturated fats: olive oil, nuts and seeds, oily fish (omega-3)

→ high in dietary fibre: wholegrains, pulses, nuts and seeds

→ moderate amount of meat, mainly unprocessed and lean

→ moderate amount of fish

→ moderate amount of dairy products

→ moderate consumption of alcohol

→ low in ultra-processed foods

→ low in saturated fat.

3 Vegetarian & vegan diets

These plant-based diets can be very gut-friendly, but the type of plants matters. And because plant-based diets exclude some food groups, it is important to make sure that all your nutritional needs are covered.

Here are a few simple principles to follow:

→ Vary the types of plants you eat, focusing on diversity.

→ Eat plenty of protein-rich foods: soy products, lentils, chickpeas (garbanzo beans), beans.

→ Make sure you get (either through food or supplements) enough key nutrients such as calcium, iron, iodine, vitamin B12, omega-3, selenium and zinc.

→ Limit ultra-processed foods full of salt, additives and preservatives.

→ Prefer wholegrains to refined grains.

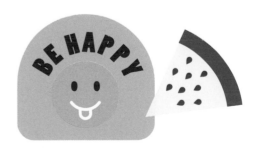

Your Checklist for
Optimal Gut Health

With so many factors influencing your gut microbiota, you might be wondering where to start. Here are some concrete tips for optimal gut health for you to experiment with.

1 Eat a balanced diet & focus on diversity

Ensure regular eating patterns with a varied range of nutritious foods (carbohydrates, proteins, healthy fats), limited amounts of highly processed food and artificial sweeteners – a bit like the Mediterranean diet. Rather than restricting your diet, make small and sustainable changes focusing on health rather than weight loss. Aim at 30 different types of plants per week (wholegrains, legumes, nuts and seeds, fruit, vegetables, herbs and spices). It is also good to eat a small amount of food rich in probiotics such as kefir, kimchi, kombucha or tempeh on a daily basis.

2 Stay hydrated & be mindful of alcohol

Increase your fluid intake as your consumption of dietary fibre goes up to avoid gut discomfort and limit your alcohol intake to a maximum of 14 units a week and no more than 2 units a day.

3 Stay active & get outside

It is good to undertake regular physical activity. Aim for 150 minutes a week of moderate intensity or 75 minutes a week of vigorous aerobic activity. Try to ensure regular exposure to the outdoors, such as in nature and reduce your exposure to smoking, unnecessary medication and pollution.

4 Protect your sleep & manage your stress

Focus on quantity of sleep (about 7–9 hours a night), as well as quality (uninterrupted) and regularity of sleep (same sleeping pattern throughout the week, in sync with daylight if possible). It is also good to notice when your stress is shifting from being a helpful motivator to a hindrance, and use tools such as meditation, yoga and exercise when needed.

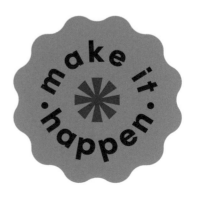

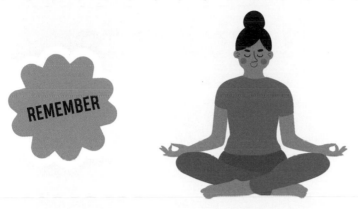

→ Eat a **balanced diet** and make sure to eat **regularly**.

→ **Focus on diversity** by aiming to eat **30 different types** of plants a week.

→ Add **fermented food** to your diet on a **daily basis**.

→ Be mindful of **alcohol** and limit your consumption.

→ Avoid restrictive diets and **focus on health** rather than weight loss.

→ **Stay hydrated** by increasing your fluid intake.

→ Work on your environment and make sure you have **regular exposure** to the outside, nature, animals and pets as well as **reducing your risk** to pollution and smoking.

→ Stay active by undertaking **regular** physical activity each week.

→ Protect your sleep and focus on **quantity, quality and regularity**.

→ **Manage your stress levels** and use tools such as meditation or yoga when needed.

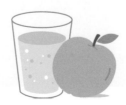

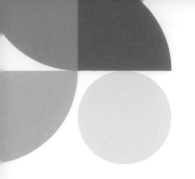

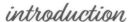

Gut
Trouble

When the gut is healthy and happy, the benefits radiate through your whole body. But unfortunately, sometimes things don't go well. Constipation, diarrhoea, bloating, nausea, fatigue, joint pain, brain fog? Your gut needs some attention.

❶ Could it be food sensitivity?

Food sensitivities are when a particular food triggers an inappropriate immune response. The immune system mistakenly thinks that the body is under threat and reacts.

This is what happens with:

→ Coeliac disease – in the presence of the protein gluten, the immune system starts attacking the small intestine and damages the gut wall.

→ Food allergies (e.g. cow's milk, nuts, soy, egg, shellfish) – when eaten, the culprit food triggers an almost instant reaction (itching, swelling of the tongue, rash, digestive symptoms, or full-blown anaphylactic reaction).

With food sensitivity, the only strategy is avoidance of the food. This might not be so crucial for people with mild pollen-food syndrome (a common food allergy in adults), but for people with severe allergies it is a matter of life or death. Luckily, food sensitivities are rare. Coeliac affects only 1 per cent of the population, while less than 4 per cent suffers from allergies.

❷ Maybe food intolerance?

In the case of food intolerance, the immune system is not involved. It's 'just' an abnormal reaction to a food in the gut, and symptoms usually appear a few hours after eating it. No harm is done to the gut itself, but the symptoms can be very debilitating: explosive poop, constant diarrhoea, tummy cramps, bloating or wind.

The main culprits for food intolerance are lactose (found in some dairy products), wheat and/or gluten, food additives, histamine, sulphite, caffeine, FODMAPs (more on these on page 51). With food intolerance, the dose matters – small amounts might be completely fine and the symptoms will only appear when the quantity eaten goes over a certain threshold.

Because of the delayed reaction, the range of possible offenders and the threshold of tolerance, it can be really challenging to pinpoint the culprit food. There are lots of 'food intolerance tests' – sadly, none is reliable. The only sensible approach is an elimination-reintroduction protocol to investigate gut symptoms. Getting support from a specialist dietitian may be particularly valuable.

❸ Or is it something else?

You might be tempted to blame a specific food for your gut symptoms, but in many cases, the problem is actually elsewhere. Stress and restrictive diets are well known to cause gut troubles, certainly as much as foods do. You might see great improvements through meditation, yoga and lifestyle change. So, before arbitrarily eliminating whole food groups from your diet, you might want to explore other avenues first.

Identifying food sensitivities

How to identify if it's a food sensitivity
A specific food triggers an immune response.

How to diagnose a food sensitivity
There are several ways to diagnose if it's a food sensitivity, such as a blood test (IgE allergies and Coeliac), prick test (IgE allergies) or elimination diet (non-IgE allergies)

Treatment
For food sensitivities, avoidance of the triggering food is required.

Common culprits
These foods may trigger a food sensitivity: egg, wheat, soy, nuts, seeds, fish, seafood, cow's milk, gluten (for Coeliac).

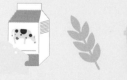

Identifying food intolerance

How to identify if it's a food intolerance
Gut reaction to certain food ingested.

How to diagnose a food intolerance
The main way to diagnose a food intolerance is to eliminate foods, then slowly reintroduce them and monitor any symptoms.

Treatment
For food intolerance, slowly reintroduce the affected food and you may find that you can tolerate a certain level before you start getting symptoms.

Common culprits
These foods may trigger a food intolerance: lactose (from dairy products), wheat, gluten, fructose, histamine, sulphites, caffeine and FODMAP (non-digestible, fermentable carbohydrates).

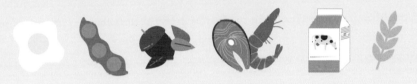

Understanding
Irritable Bowel Syndrome

Irritable bowel syndrome (IBS) is a very common condition – it affects
10 per cent of the population, mainly women (two-thirds of IBS sufferers).
It is considered a 'functional' gastrointestinal disorder because the gut
appears otherwise normal, but it can make your life miserable. Luckily,
there are a few things you can do to keep your symptoms under control.

1 Is it IBS?

Frustratingly, there is no specific test for IBS. It is diagnosed by default, once other gut diseases have been ruled out – diseases like Coeliac, Crohn's disease and ulcerative colitis.

The symptoms are very much like the ones of food intolerance:

→ issues with bowel movements (diarrhoea, constipation, urgency)

→ abdominal pain, cramps, bloating, wind

→ lethargy, backache, nausea.

In fact, people with IBS often present with food intolerances, but it is actually more than that.

2 What's going on?

IBS is a disorder of the gut-brain axis caused by an oversensitive gut. In IBS, the communication between the brain and the gut is dialled up to the max:

→ Signals emitted by the gut microbiome trigger exaggerated responses from the brain.

→ Signals from the brain drastically affect digestion and the gut microbiota's activity.

You can get stuck in a relentless feedback loop: the brain receives a signal of discomfort from the gut. It triggers a stress response, which creates an urge to go to the loo. The urge is so intense that it amps up the feeling of anxiety, etc. You get the gist! Reassuringly, IBS doesn't cause lasting damage to the gut, and it doesn't lead to serious bowel conditions like colitis or cancer. Still, it can take a serious toll on your quality of life.

3 First steps

Before considering the drastic step of completely transforming your diet by cutting out large food groups, there are a few powerful actions you can take:

→ Go for smaller meals, eating more frequently.

→ Take your time to chew your food.

→ Don't skip meals and avoid eating late at night.

→ Reduce caffeine and carbonated drinks.

→ Stay hydrated throughout the day.

→ Avoid too much fat and too much spicy and ultra-processed food.

→ Limit fresh fruit to 3 portions a day (and avoid fruit juices and smoothies).

→ Move your body.

→ Protect your sleep.

→ Learn to manage your stress.

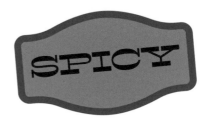

Symptoms you shouldn't ignore

Even if you suspect irritable bowel syndrome (IBS), it is a good idea to go to your doctor to rule out any other conditions – especially if you present with the following symptoms:

→ **Unintentional weight loss**
→ **Blood in your stools**

LOW FODMAP DIET?

If the tips listed above aren't enough, you might want to look at your diet. It is possible that some FODMAP foods are the cause of your trouble. FODMAP stands for Fermentable Oligosaccharides, Disaccharides, Monosaccharides and Polyols. These are carbohydrates that aren't well absorbed in the small intestine and end up fermenting in the large intestine. For most people this fermentation process is harmless, but for people with a hyper-sensitive gut, the gut microbiota activity can cause that chain reaction of distorted signals between the brain and gut. That is why people with IBS may be recommended to follow a low-FODMAP diet.

It is important to remember that a low FODMAP diet doesn't mean exclusion of all FODMAP foods forever. Rather than a traditional diet, the low FODMAP diet is more of a protocol to help you identify which specific foods:
→ should be avoided completely
→ are tolerated when consumed in small or moderate amounts
→ are totally safe.

It is structured around three phases – restriction, reintroduction and personalisation – to make sure that only the strict minimum of food is excluded. Remember that your objective should always be to have a diet as wide and varied as possible.

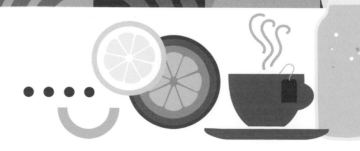

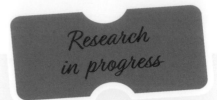

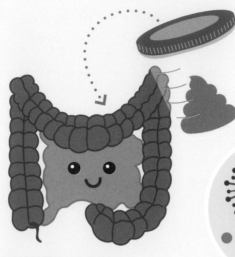

Faecal Microbiota Transplant
Searching new ways to transform the gut microbiota of sick people.

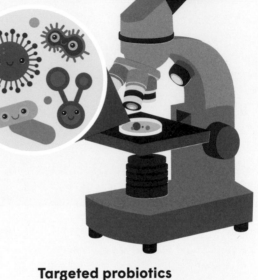

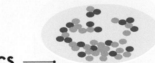

PROBIOTICS —

Targeted probiotics
Searching for the right microbes to treat specific conditions.

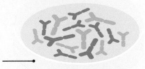

PREBIOTICS —

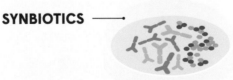

SYNBIOTICS —

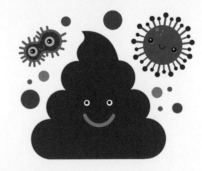

Poop test
Searching answers to health by analysing people's gut microbiota.

Synbiotics
Searching for the right combination of probiotics and prebiotics for optimal results.

Gut & Health – What's Next?

Synbiotics, psychobiotics, stool samples – the gut microbiome is a buzzing field for researchers. Medicine tomorrow might look very different. In fact, it already does!

1 Targeted probiotics

Today, most gut microbes are still being researched by scientists. Could one bacterium be helpful to fight obesity? Which strain may slow down the progression of Alzheimer's? Could you prevent depression with probiotics? Researchers are exploring thousands of microbes to identify which therapeutic benefits they might hold, but at the moment, it is still a big mystery. When using probiotics, remember that it is very much 'trial and error', with no certainty of success. Results will be linked to your use of judgement, patience and systematic trial.

2 Synbiotics

Since some specific fibres (prebiotics) are particularly loved by specific good bacteria (probiotics), how about combining the two to get the best chance for a desired health benefit? Scientists are looking for complementary pre- and probiotics to enhance both. It is early days, but in a few years' time, synbiotics might be regularly prescribed by your family doctor.

3 FMT

Faecal Microbiota Transplant (FMT) is an exciting, emerging therapy for the treatment of gut diseases. The idea is to take some of the gut microbiome from a healthy donor (from a stool sample) and to place it in the patient's gut. It might sound like science fiction, but it is already used for people suffering from severe Clostridium difficile infection, and it could soon be used for other illnesses like inflammatory bowel disease (e.g. ulcerative colitis).

4 Poop test

Most research on the gut microbiome is based on studying stool samples. You will find lots of expensive gut microbiome test kits on the internet, promising to reveal the secret of your gut. Should you get your poop tested to see if your gut is healthy or not? The answer is: no, not yet. You will get a list of all the microbes that live in your gut, but what can you do with this information? We just don't know enough yet to interpret those results.

This field is only just starting to reveal its potential and there is still a lot to understand. Watch this space.

Your Journey to a
Healthier Gut

Your gut is unique and mysterious. Look after it by feeding it rather than depriving it. And notice how it looks after you. It's a two-way relationship.

This second brain that is your gut microbiota is a powerful organ that you need to care for. But so much more needs to be understood. While scientists explore new ways to harness the gut microbiome for health, you can't go wrong by following these simple principles:

❶ Within your control

A diverse, balanced diet supports gut health, while long-term, restrictive diets could cause nutritional deficiencies and impoverish the gut microbiome.

→ Expand your diet rather than reducing it.

Food rich in dietary fibre, polyphenols and fermented foods help the gut microbiome to thrive.

→ Aim for more plant-based foods and add some fermented food to your plate.

Things other than diet also affect your gut microbiome – factors such as pollution, sleep, stress, physical activity, medication, environment and relationship with food.

→ Think beyond diet and see how your lifestyle impacts your gut health.

❷ When help is needed

When the gut is struggling, it is important to know what is going on to choose the right strategy. Is it an allergy? An intolerance? An issue with your gut-brain communication? Or something completely different? The gut is connected to so many health aspects that it can be hard to pinpoint precisely what needs to be done to soothe your gut and your body.

Don't fall for magic pills, food intolerance tests or your neighbour's advice, which all might be counterproductive.

Always check with a healthcare professional to get a proper diagnosis, and explore more avenues than just diet.

This book is packed with ideas and recipes to feed your gut and its residents. Try them out, get inspired and create your own gut-friendly diet. Your journey to a healthier gut begins here!

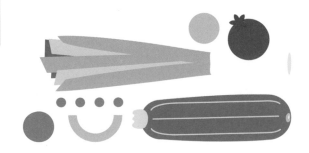

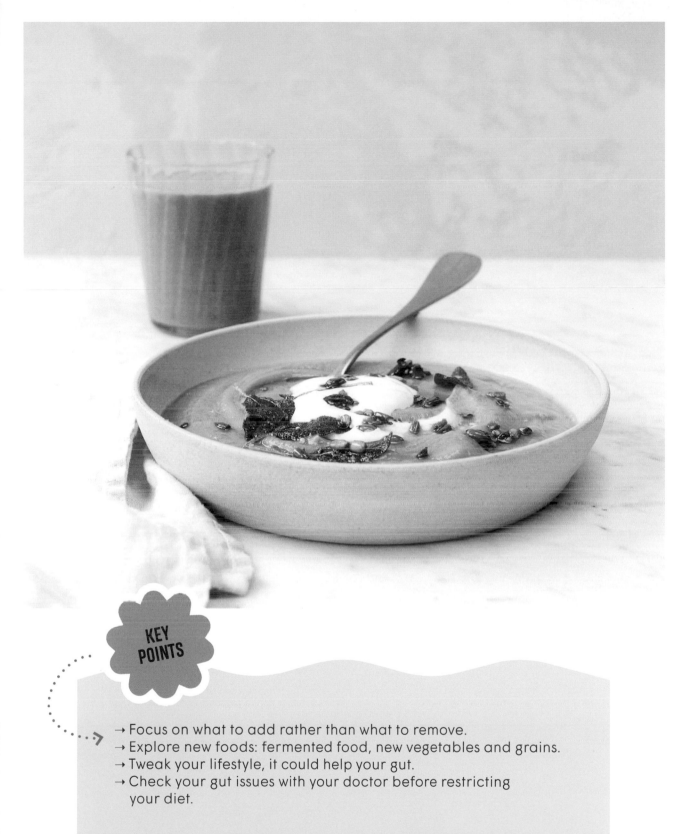

KEY POINTS

→ Focus on what to add rather than what to remove.
→ Explore new foods: fermented food, new vegetables and grains.
→ Tweak your lifestyle, it could help your gut.
→ Check your gut issues with your doctor before restricting your diet.

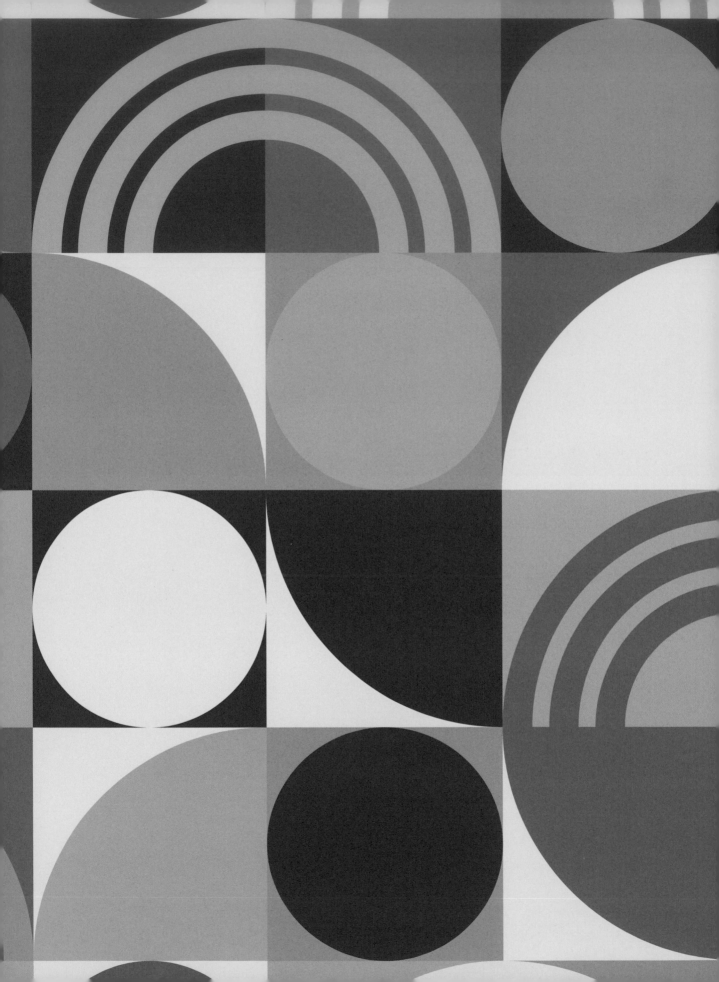

Basic
Recipes

WITH

- Ingredients you need to cook healthy recipes
- How to make kimchi & lacto-fermented pickles
- How to make live yoghurt
- How to sprout seeds & pulses easily

Storecupboard ingredients

It can be difficult to know what to eat to support your gut, but the reality is that many of the foods we already have in the cupboard are ingredients that can be considered the basis of a gut-healthy diet. Pulses, grains, nuts, seeds and spices offer fibre, which can help support our digestive system, as well as prebiotics and other important nutrients.

Pulses & grains

Pulses and grains are staples in diets all over the world. Pulses are a great source of protein, healthy carbohydrates, several vitamins, calcium, zinc and potassium. They offer an excellent nutrition package and help to stabilise blood sugar, preventing and managing type 2 diabetes. They are also powerful antioxidants and have anti-inflammatory properties. Whole grains offer a complete package of health benefits, unlike refined ones. It is good to plan ahead and cook pulses and grains, then freeze them in batches.

Nuts & seeds

Nuts and seeds are packed with micronutrients and healthy fats. They can help keep you fuller for longer and are among the best sources of plant-based proteins. It is always handy to keep a good selection in your pantry as quick snacks or as enhancers to different recipes.

Spices

Spices play a significant role in the way we cook and consume food. They provide a depth of flavour to any dish and are known to have several health benefits.

Flours

Flour is a pantry staple used for both savoury and sweet recipes. Some are healthier than others and it is good to replace white flour with more wholesome options. Interestingly, some flours aren't actually made from grains but from nuts or seeds, such as almond, buckwheat, quinoa and linseeds (flax seeds).

Oil

The health benefits of extra virgin olive oil are unequalled, from its anti-inflammatory properties to reduction of heart and diabetes problems. It is the cornerstone of the Mediterranean diet and is naturally high in healthy fatty acids. Rapeseed oil is a great source of some omega-3 fats and as it has a high smoke point, it makes it a good choice for frying or roasting.

Condiments

Kimchi, pickle and pesto are only a few examples of adding condiments to your meals to enhance flavour and also add health benefits.

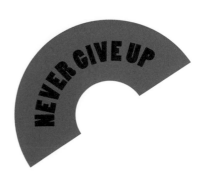

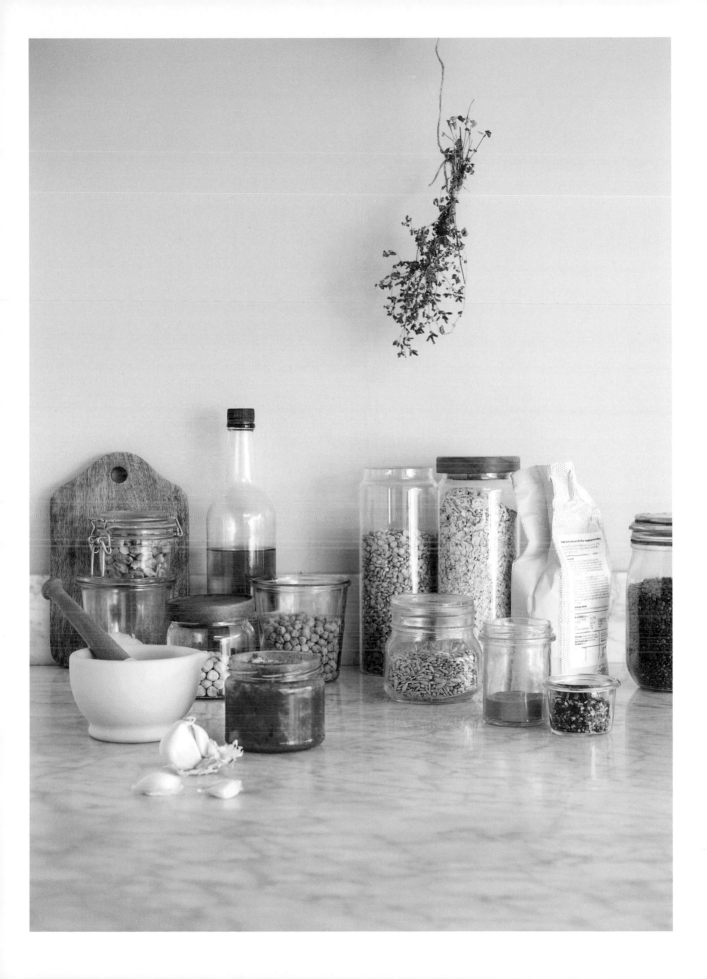

Protein &
dairy products

Research shows that certain types of foods, in particular the ones rich in fibre, can help the microbes in the gut to flourish best, but a balanced diet needs to include protein-rich foods. For example, live yoghurt contains beneficial probiotics; beans and pulses are filled with prebiotics and fibre, which are important for overall digestion; and tempeh and tofu are perfect plant-based protein to eat for your gut as an alternative to meat.

Egg

Eggs are an important and versatile ingredient for cooking. They are rich in nutrients, including proteins, vitamins and minerals. The yolk contains fat-soluble vitamins (such as vitamins D and E) and essential fatty acids, while most of the protein is found in the egg white.

Fish

Fish is an easy and nutritious way to add vitamins and minerals to your diet and makes a great high-protein alternative to red meat and poultry. It is recommended to eat at least one portion per week of oily fish, such as salmon, mackerel, anchovies or sardines, as they contain omega-3 fats.

Meat

A healthy balanced diet can include protein from meat such as chicken, lamb and beef. When buying meat you should always go for the leanest option.

Pulses

Pulses are also an important plant-based source of protein. The amount of protein in lentils, beans, chickpeas (garbanzo beans) and peas is 2–3 times the levels found in grains like quinoa, oats or barley.

Tofu

Soy products, like tofu, are powerful antioxidants. Tofu is a popular plant-based meat and dairy alternative and a rich source of protein, providing all nine essential amino acids we need for growth, repair and functions like immunity. It also contains vitamins and minerals including calcium as well as beneficial isoflavones or phytoestrogens (page 35). It can be cooked in many different ways, from stir-fries to marinated and baked.

Tempeh

Made from fermented soy beans, tempeh is a nutrient-dense, plant-based ingredient rich in protein, which is also known for its filling and satiating effect. It is rich in fibre, the type known to be prebiotic, that feeds the beneficial bacteria in the gut. It is higher in protein than tofu, and is less processed. Tempeh is very versatile in cooking: add it to stir-fries with vegetables and brown rice, marinate it, fry it and add it to your favourite bowl recipe.

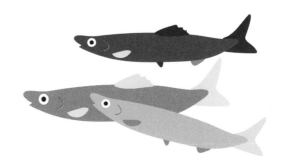

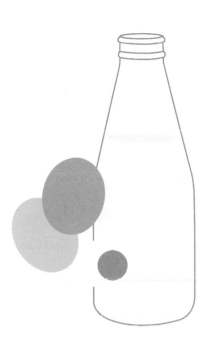

Milk, cheese & yoghurt

Dairy products like milk, cheese and yoghurt are rich in protein and contain many essential vitamins and minerals, including calcium and magnesium, as well as supplying all the essential amino acids that our body needs. Regular yoghurt consumption can help to improve gut bacteria and decrease symptoms of lactose intolerance. It is always best to opt for natural, unsweetened yoghurt that is made just from milk and contains live bacteria, which are sometimes called 'starter cultures'. Additionally, to reap the gut health benefits, make sure the label reads: 'contains live active cultures'.

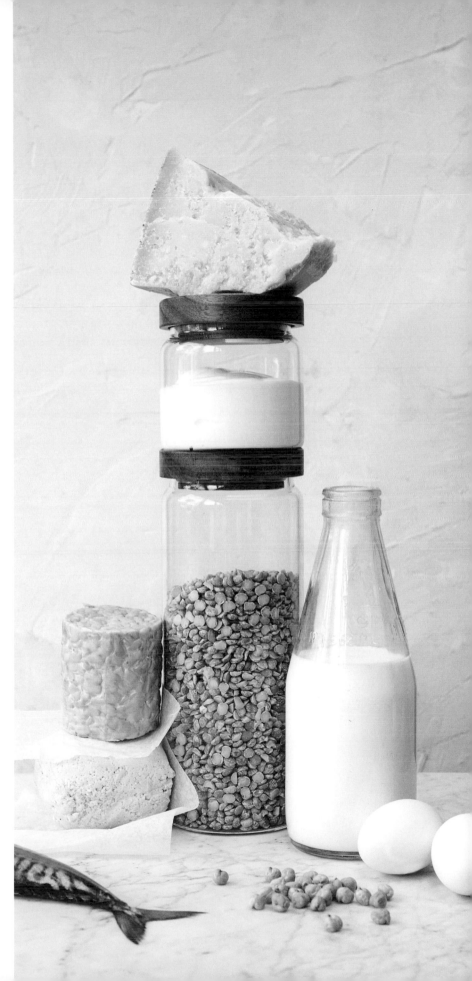

Fruit
& vegetables

The easiest way to ensure a healthy gut is by eating plenty of fruit and vegetables that are high in fibre and promote a proper intestinal balance. Vegetables are the best source of nutrients for a healthy gut microbiome. Soups are a great way to consume multiple servings of vegetables at once, and because the leafy greens wilt easily and reduce in size, they are the perfect vegetables for tossing into pasta and making sauces.

Bananas

Bananas are high in fibre, which can help keep you feeling fuller for longer, lower cholesterol and may reduce bloating. As they contain a prebiotic fibre, bananas can help to feed your gut's bacteria to improve digestive health and boost your immune system. One medium banana provides approximately 10 per cent of a person's fibre needs for a day. Bananas are also rich in potassium, which may lower blood pressure and protect against heart disease.

Berries

Berries, like blueberries, blackberries and raspberries, are among the healthiest foods we can eat to help diversify our gut bacteria. They contain high levels of antioxidants, which may protect our cells from free radical damage, as well as enough plentiful fibre, which may increase the feeling of fullness. Berries are also low in calories but rich in lots of vitamins and minerals like vitamin C and manganese.

Other fruits

Kiwi fruit is a fat-free, nutrient-dense source of energy. The skin of pears contains 3–4 times as many phenolic phytonutrients, like antioxidants, anti-inflammatory and anti-cancer, as the flesh. Apples are an incredibly nutritious fruit that offers multiple health benefits, rich in fibre and antioxidants. They can also reduce the risk of many chronic conditions such as diabetes, heart disease and cancer and improve gut and brain health.

Leafy greens

Leafy greens, such as spinach, kale and silverbeet (Swiss chard), play an important role in a healthy diet. They are excellent sources of fibre, packed with different types of vitamins and minerals, including vitamin K, iron and calcium, but are also low in calories. A diet rich in leafy greens can offer numerous health benefits including a reduced risk of obesity, heart disease and high blood pressure.

Brassicas

Most vegetables are naturally high in fibre, but the brassica or cruciferous family, such as broccoli and cauliflower, gets a gold star. They also contain high levels of carotenoid, vitamins C and K, folate, manganese and potassium. When shopping, avoid any vegetable that shows signs of ageing and always choose the crispest and greenest type. It is also important not to overcook brassicas in order not to lose all their benefits.

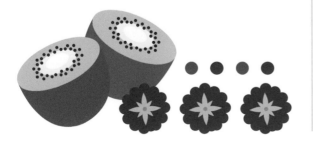

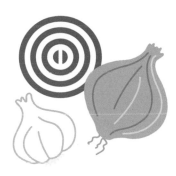

Garlic, onions & leeks

Garlic, onions, leeks and French shallots stimulate the growth of beneficial microbiota. Due to its antibacterial, antifungal and antiviral properties, garlic is known to reduce inflammation and lower high blood pressure, while onions can normalise digestion and leeks are rich in antioxidants and sulphur compounds. Leeks are also a good source of soluble fibre, which feeds the beneficial bacteria in your gut, and these bacteria reduce inflammation and promote digestive health.

Potatoes & Jerusalem artichokes

Also high on the prebiotic list is the resistant starch found in potatoes or Jerusalem artichokes, while artichokes, chicory (endive), asparagus and carrots are rich in polyphenols.

Herbs

Herbs, like spices, can elevate dishes from dull to delicious and it turns out that they are also important for gut health. They can help with digestive function and support the gut's ability to break down food. Herbs such as clove, rosemary, sage, oregano and peppermint are excellent sources of antioxidants with their high content of phenolic compounds (see page 35).

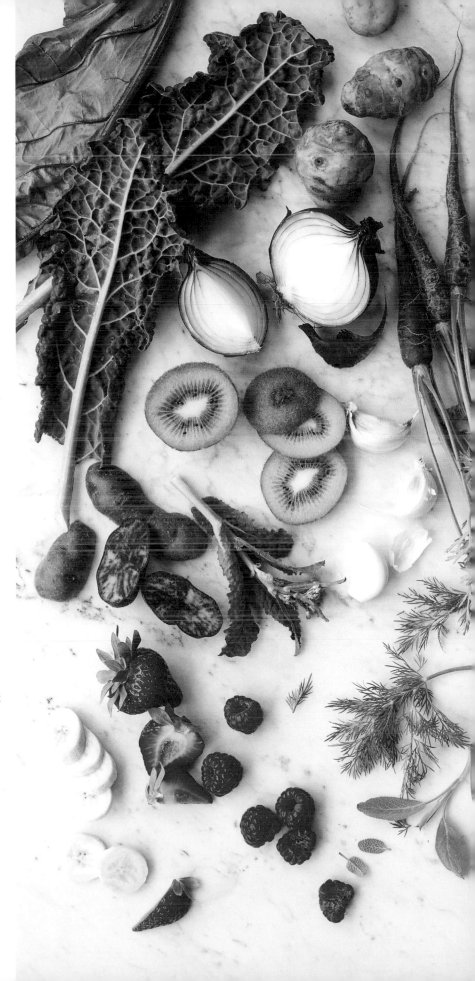

Classic Kimchi

Kimchi is the national food of South Korea. It is crunchy and flavoursome, and with its vitamins, minerals and antioxidants, it can provide impressive health benefits. As with all fermented food, kimchi is an excellent probiotic and contains the same Lactobacilli bacteria found in yoghurt and other fermented foods. Spicy and sour, kimchi can be eaten by itself or used in cooking to flavour stews, noodles and salads – just add it after cooking to preserve its good bacteria.

MAKES: 750 G (1 LB 11 OZ)
PREPARATION: 6 DAYS
COOK: 0 MINUTES

1 large Chinese cabbage, quartered
  and chopped to desired thickness
60 g (2 oz) sea salt
100 g (3½ oz) carrot, grated
1 bunch spring (green) onions, cut
  into 2.5 cm (1 in) slices
100 g (3½ oz) daikon radish, peeled
  and cut into matchsticks
1 tablespoon soy sauce
½ tablespoon grated garlic
1 teaspoon grated ginger
1 teaspoon chilli powder
1 teaspoon paprika

Put cabbage and salt into a large bowl and massage the salt into the cabbage. Cover with 2 litres (8 cups) water and leave to soak overnight. Next day, drain and rinse cabbage a few times to get rid of excess salt, then squeeze out any water and put into a large bowl. Add all remaining ingredients and mix well. Transfer mixture to a sterilised 1 litre (34 fl oz) jar, pressing down firmly until liquid rises to cover vegetables. Seal jar with lid and leave it to ferment for 5 days. Taste kimchi once a day, opening jar and pressing vegetables down to keep them covered with liquid. Once it has reached your preferred flavour, transfer to a sterilised smaller jar, squash down well, seal with a lid and chill in fridge for up to 9 months. You can eat it immediately, but it is better to leave it for another 2 weeks to allow flavours to develop.

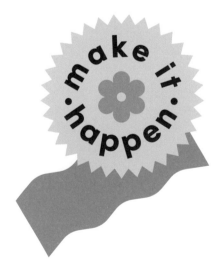

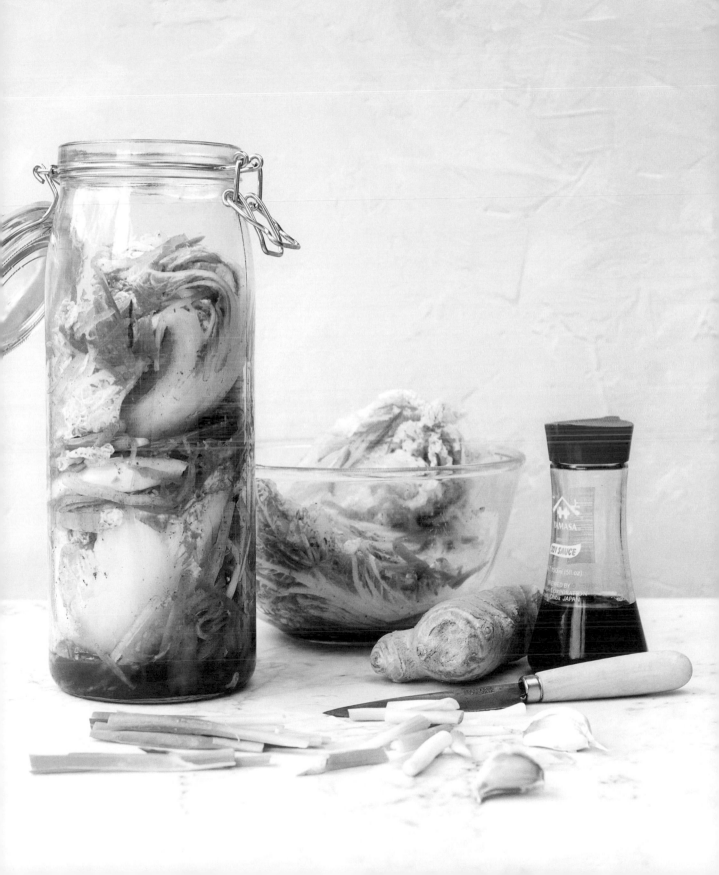

Live Yoghurt

Live yoghurt has been fermented with live cultures or friendly bacteria that are considered good for the digestive system. It contains nearly every nutrient that your body needs and also high amounts of calcium, which helps with the health of your teeth and bones. Help to balance the natural bacteria in your gut by trying to regularly include live yoghurt into your diet: add it to fresh fruit in the morning, dollop it in soup or use it as an ingredient in baking.

MAKES: 375 ML (1½ CUPS)
PREPARATION: 13 HOURS
COOK: 15 MINUTES

500 ml (2 cups) full-fat milk
50 g (1¾ oz) natural yoghurt

Pour milk into a very clean saucepan and bring to the boil. Lower heat slightly and simmer for 15 minutes, stirring constantly, until milk is reduced by a quarter. Pour milk into a sterilised glass container, leave to cool to 45°C (113°F), then stir in yoghurt. Cover with a plate and leave in a cold oven, with the light on, for 8–12 hours. Remove from the oven to cool before storing in the fridge for up to a week.

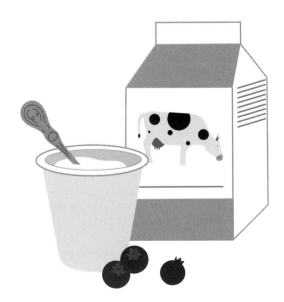

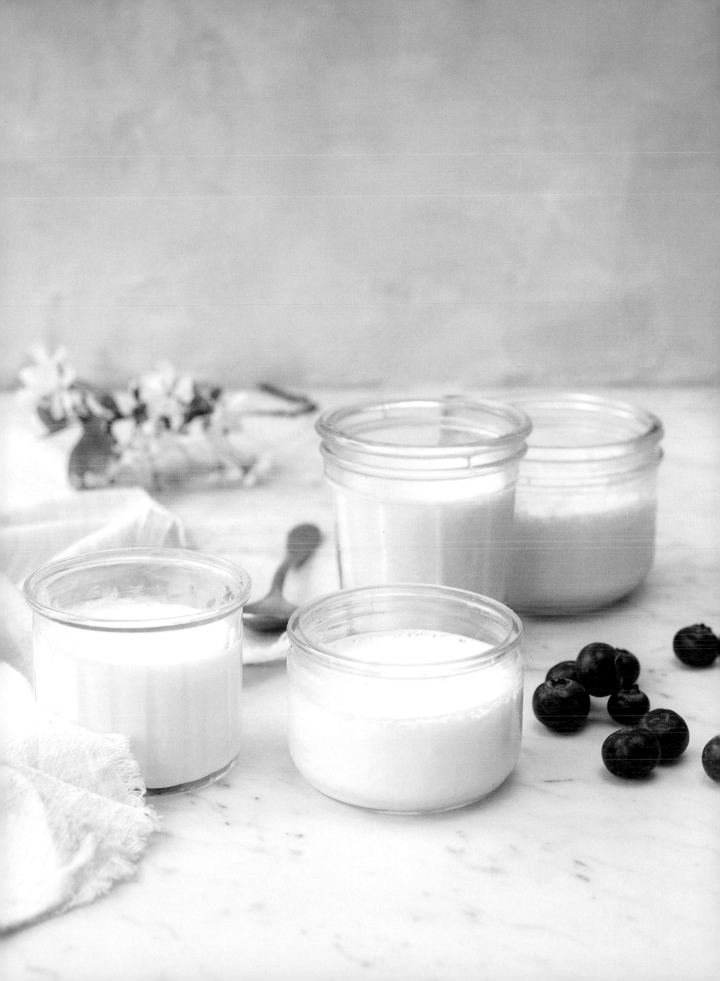

Sprouting Seeds & Pulses

Recently, the process of sprouting has become more popular and this is because eating sprouted seeds, pulses or grains, unlocks vital benefits. Sprouts contain vitamins C, B and proteins, and the process breaks down enzyme inhibitors so the body can easily absorb minerals. Their firm, crunchy texture is good for stir-fries as well as salads, as a topping for dips, broths or as a sprinkle on top of a bowl of noodles. Only use seeds, lentils or beans that are intended for sprouting, and if your sprouts go brown or have a sour smell, then discard them. Make sure all your equipment, including your jars, are sterilised before using.

MAKES: 50 G (1¾ OZ)
PREPARATION: 7 DAYS
COOK: 45 MINUTES

50 g (1¾ oz) alfalfa, broccoli, dried peas, lentils or chickpeas (garbanzo beans), specifically for home sprouting

Rinse and drain seeds or pulses, then put them into a clean mason jar, cover with 150 ml (5 fl oz) cool water and stir to make sure all seeds are wet. Cover top with a piece of muslin (cheesecloth) secured with an elastic band or string and leave to soak overnight at room temperature. Next morning, using a sieve, strain seeds or pulses, then rinse and drain seeds or pulses again and put back into jar. To remove all excess water, put jar upside down in a bowl at a 45-degree angle to drain. Repeat same process in evening, then again for next 5 days, or until you get sprout length you want. Rinse sprouts again, drain and pat dry before putting them into an airtight sterilised jar ready to be stored in fridge. For pulses, simmer for 45 minutes before doing same process as for seeds. Store in fridge for up to 5 days.

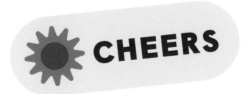
CHEERS

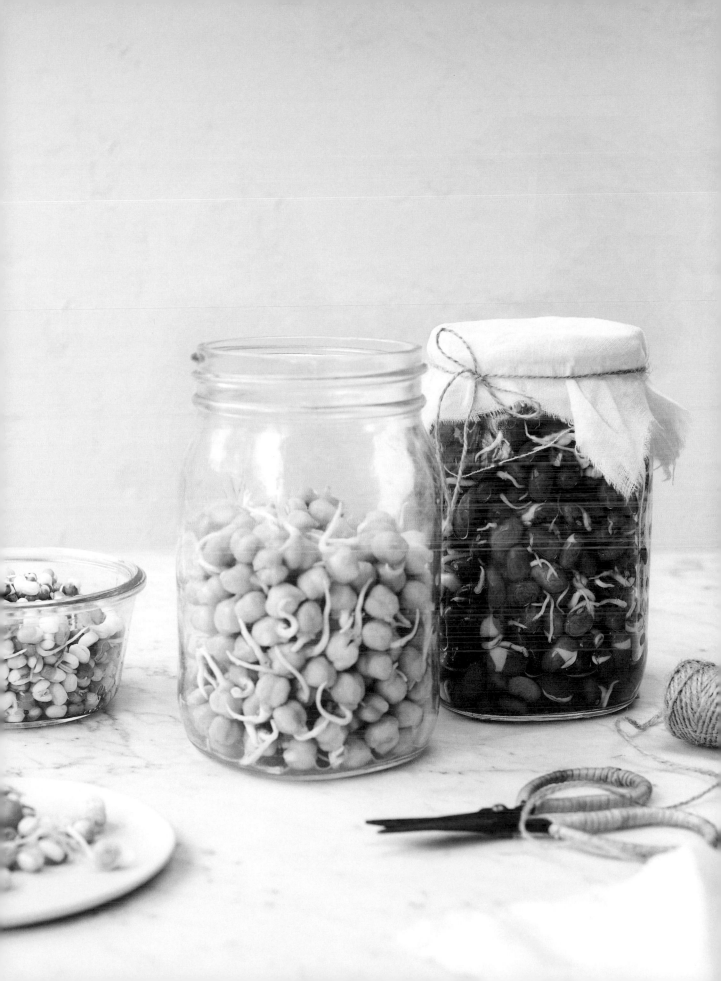

Triple Nut Butter

Nuts are low in carbohydrates and loaded with heart-healthy monounsaturated fats. They also have plenty of nutrients, such as vitamin E, magnesium and potassium, as well as selenium and manganese. A serving of nut butter is a great source of valuable nutrients. Homemade nut butter is easy to make and allows you to create your own blends. Nut butter is a versatile ingredient, you can stir it into porridge, use it as a base for muffins or cakes, add it to smoothies, spread it on toast, eat it with fresh fruit for an additional nutrient punch, or stir it into sauces for added flavour.

MAKES: 600 G (1 LB 5 OZ)
PREPARATION: 5 MINUTES
COOK: 12 MINUTES

450 g (1 lb) mixed almonds, walnuts, hazelnuts
100 ml (3½ fl oz) coconut oil, melted
3 Medjool dates, stoned
pinch of salt

Preheat oven to 190°C (375°F). Arrange nuts on a lined baking tray in a single layer and bake for 12 minutes. Remove and leave to cool completely. Blitz nuts with oil, dates and salt in a blender, stopping to scrape down as necessary, until mixture is completely smooth. If it is too dry add some water. Store in an airtight glass container in fridge for up to 3 weeks.

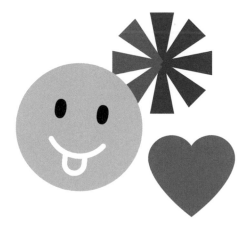

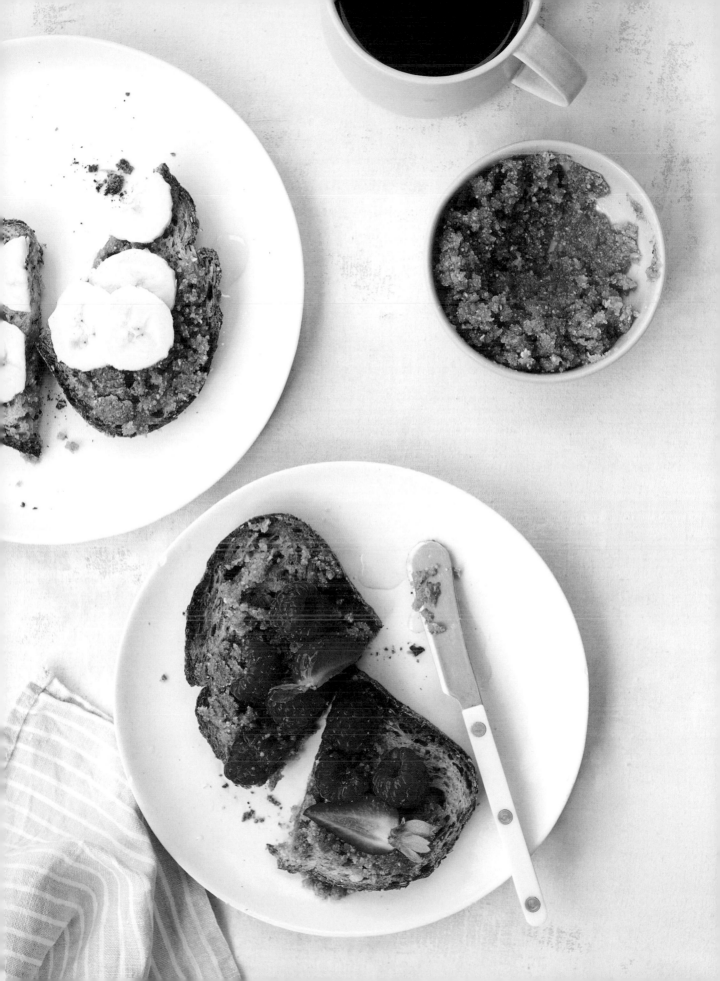

Super Seedy & Multigrain Granola

Granola is a very popular breakfast ingredient. While store-bought ones may be cheaper, making your own gives you control on prioritising wholegrains rather than refined sugar and palm oil. Wholegrains, such as oats, contain prebiotic fibre, which may increase the levels of healthy gut bacteria compared to cereals made with refined grains. This homemade version is full of protein-rich nuts and seeds as well as a small amount of honey and salt. There are plenty of ways to enjoy granola from sprinkling it onto yoghurt or ice cream, baking with it or eating it as a snack.

MAKES: 575 G (1 LB 4 OZ)
PREPARATION: 5 MINUTES
COOK: 20 MINUTES

150 g (5½ oz) jumbo oats
150 g (5½ oz) grain of choice
    (spelt, barley, rye)
80 g (2¾ oz) mixed seeds
80 g (2¾ oz) mixed nuts, roughly
    chopped
3 tablespoons coconut oil
50 ml (1¾ fl oz) honey
pinch of salt
20 g (⅓ cup) coconut flakes

Preheat oven to 150°C (300°F). Put oats, grain, mixed seeds and nuts into a large bowl and mix well to combine. Heat oil and honey together in a small pan for 1 minute, whisking thoroughly. Pour over the dry ingredients and stir to coat evenly. Spread mix out on a lined baking tray and bake for 10 minutes. Add coconut flakes and bake for another 10 minutes. Leave to cool before transferring to an airtight container. Store for up to 2 weeks.

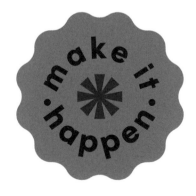

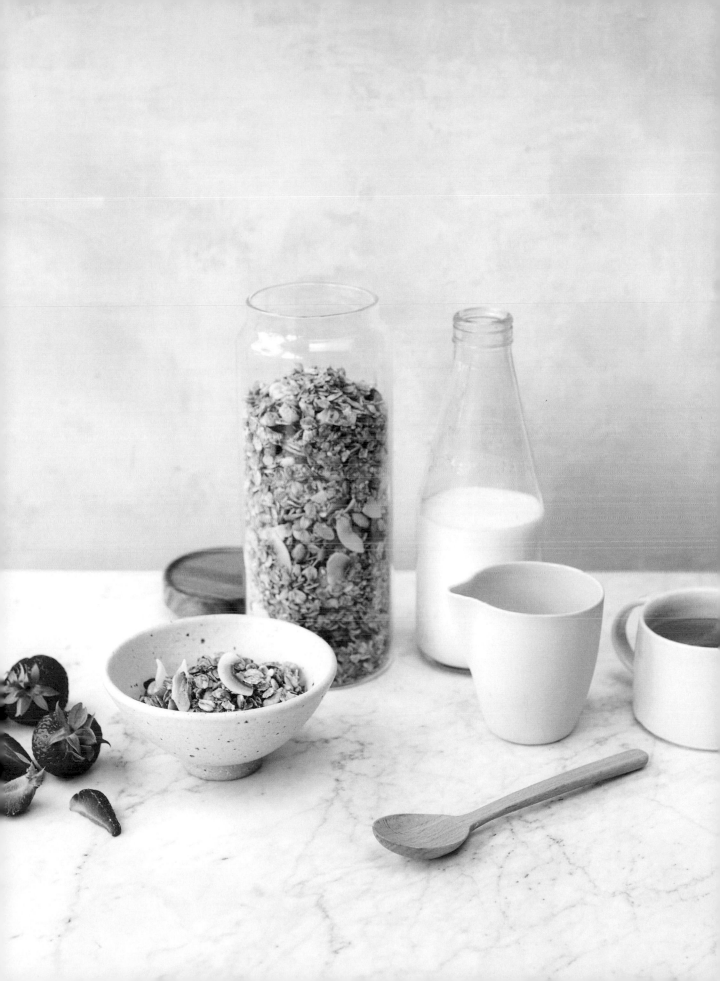

Lacto-fermented Pickles

Lacto-fermentation is a type of fermentation that uses lactic-acid-producing bacteria to preserve foods while adding flavour, texture and aroma. It is a process that increases the nutritional value of food and makes vegetables easier to digest. It is also rich in nutrients and good for the microbiota. Every vegetable can be fermented, and they are perfect for snacking on or adding to a meal for a probiotic boost as well as a flavour enhancer.

MAKES: 500 G (1 LB 2 OZ)
PREPARATION: 2 DAYS
COOK: 0 MINUTES

500 g (1 lb 2 oz) carrot, broccoli, radish or cucumber
15 g (½ oz) sea salt
¼ teaspoon black peppercorns
1 bay leaf
1 garlic clove, chopped

Wash a 1 litre (34 fl oz) mason jar with hot soapy water and rinse well. Chop or slice vegetables of your choice. Put salt and 375 ml (1½ cups) water into a large bowl and stir until salt has dissolved. Put all vegetables, peppercorns, bay leaf and garlic into the clean jar, pour in salty water and press down with a clean rolling pin until juice comes to top, leaving about 2 cm (¾ in). Add more water, if necessary, to cover vegetables. Make sure vegetables are submerged. Cover jar tightly with lid and leave to stand at room temperature for 2 days. After 2 days, open jar to taste pickles and to release gases produced during fermentation. When pickles taste to your liking, transfer jar to fridge and eat within a month.

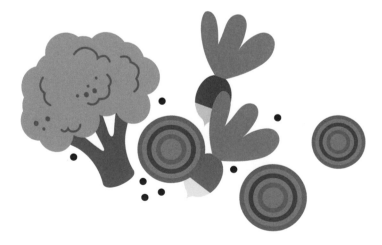

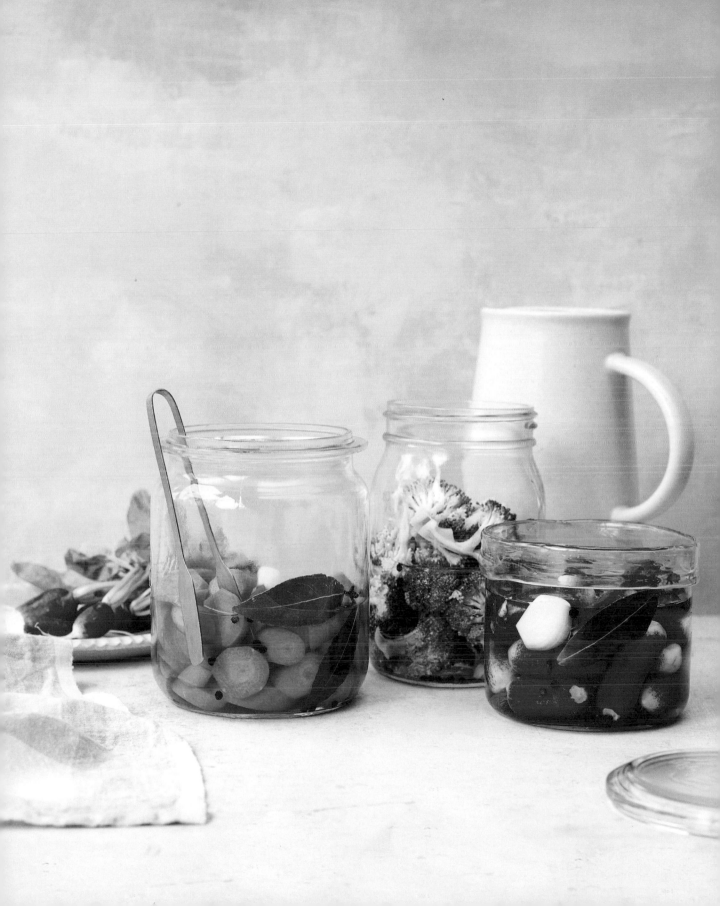

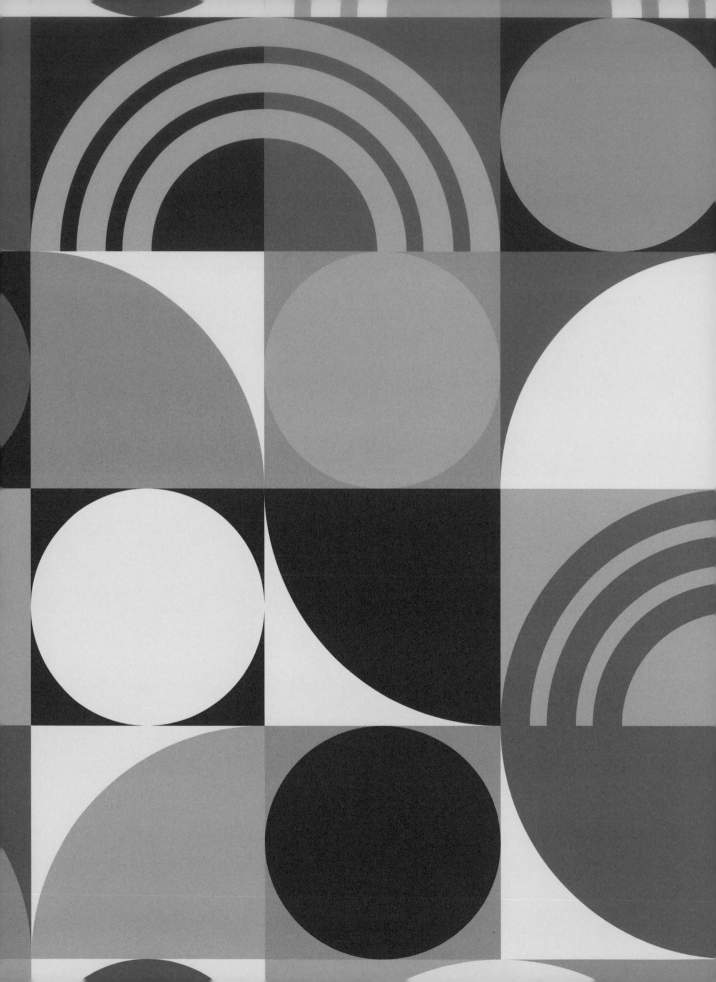

28 days
Recipes

WITH

- A weekly shopping list for a whole month
- Menus for each day of the week for a month
- 3 recipes for each day of the week to help improve your gut health

My shopping list

Fruit

- ○ 1 kiwi fruit
- ○ 1 banana
- ○ 75 g (2¾ oz) raspberries or pitted cherries
- ○ 150 g (1 cup) blueberries
- ○ 1 grapefruit
- ○ 100 g (3½ oz) mixed fresh fruit
- ○ 150 g (1 cup) strawberries
- ○ 150 g (5½ oz) mixed melon
- ○ 30 g (1 oz) grapes
- ○ 1 orange
- ○ 50 ml (1¾ fl oz) orange juice
- ○ 3 tbsp lime juice + 1 lime wedge
- ○ 2 tbsp lemon juice + 1 lemon wedge
- ○ 1 tsp grated lemon zest

Vegetables

- ○ 3½ red onions
- ○ 4 garlic cloves
- ○ 200 g (7 oz) spinach
- ○ 150 g (5½ oz) mixed mushrooms
- ○ 1½ fennel bulbs
- ○ ½ small winter cabbage
- ○ 150 g (5½ oz) heirloom tomatoes
- ○ 2 tomatoes + 2 medium tomatoes
- ○ 5 cherry tomatoes
- ○ 1½ avocados
- ○ 50 g (1¾ oz) baby rocket (arugula)
- ○ 50 g (1¾ oz) watercress
- ○ 60 g (2 oz) cavolo nero
- ○ 8 small carrots
- ○ 2 zucchini (courgettes), 1 yellow and 1 green
- ○ 50 g (1¾ oz) soffritto (red onion, celery, carrot)
- ○ 2 cm (¾ in) piece + 2 tsp grated fresh ginger
- ○ 2 tbsp coriander (cilantro)
- ○ 2 tbsp parsley
- ○ 1 tsp chives
- ○ 2 tbsp basil
- ○ 1 rosemary sprig
- ○ 1 tsp mint
- ○ 20 g (¾ oz) mixed herbs (basil, parsley, mint)
- ○ Handful kale leaves
- ○ Baby salad leaves

Fridge Products

- ○ 150 g (5½ oz) skin-on salmon fillet
- ○ 2 mackerel fillets
- ○ 2 bone-in chicken thighs
- ○ 50 g (1¾ oz) tempeh
- ○ 2 tbsp kimchi
- ○ 600 ml (20½ fl oz) vegetable stock

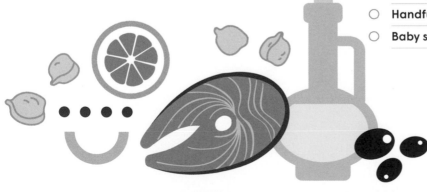

In the Storecupboard

- ○ 1 slice sourdough bread
- ○ 80 g (2¾ oz) pappardelle pasta
- ○ 50 g (1¾ oz) cooked brown rice
- ○ 125 g (4½ oz) Instant polenta
- ○ 280 g (10 oz) green or brown lentils
- ○ 50 g (1¾ oz) canned borlotti (cranberry) beans
- ○ 240 g (8½ oz) canned chickpeas (garbanzo beans)
- ○ 100 g (3½ oz) canned cannellini beans
- ○ 400 ml (13½ fl oz) can coconut milk
- ○ 100 g (3½ oz) spelt
- ○ 2 tbsp oats
- ○ 45 g (1½ oz) granola
- ○ 45 g (1½ oz) cashew nut butter
- ○ 3½ tbsp mixed toasted nuts
- ○ 1 tsp toasted pumpkin seeds
- ○ 10 black olives
- ○ 1 tsp salted capers
- ○ rye flour
- ○ wholemeal (whole-wheat) flour
- ○ baking powder
- ○ extra virgin olive oil
- ○ balsamic vinegar
- ○ maple syrup
- ○ honey
- ○ harissa paste
- ○ garam masala
- ○ poppy seeds
- ○ ground turmeric
- ○ paprika
- ○ chilli flakes
- ○ saffron threads

Eggs & Dairy Products

- ○ 100 ml (3½ fl oz) kefir milk
- ○ 1 tbsp full-fat milk
- ○ 180 g (¾ cup) live yoghurt
- ○ 200 g (7 oz) Greek yoghurt
- ○ 100 g (3½ oz) labneh
- ○ 50 g (1¾ oz) Taleggio cheese
- ○ 25 g (1 oz) parmesan
- ○ 80 g (2¾ oz) feta
- ○ 100 g (3½ oz) ricotta
- ○ 55 g (2 oz) butter
- ○ 5 large eggs

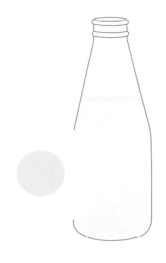

Monday

A delicious and super healthy way to start the week, the kefir smoothie loaded with probiotics and superfoods, is naturally sweet and made without added sugars.

Breakfast

BALANCE KEFIR SMOOTHIE

SERVES: 1
PREPARATION: 5 MINUTES
COOK: 0 MINUTES

1 kiwi fruit
1 banana
75 g (2¾ oz) raspberries or pitted cherries
2 tablespoons oats
100 ml (3½ fl oz) kefir milk
50 ml (1¾ fl oz) orange juice

Peel and slice kiwi fruit and banana. Put into a blender with remaining ingredients and blend until smooth. Serve immediately.

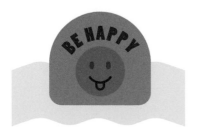

Lunch

TURMERIC & COCONUT DAHL

SERVES: 4
PREPARATION: 5 MINUTES
COOK: 30 MINUTES

2 tablespoons extra virgin olive oil
1 red onion, finely diced
2 cm (¾ in) piece ginger, peeled and grated
1 teaspoon ground turmeric
2 teaspoons garam masala
200 g (7 oz) brown or green lentils
400 ml (13½ fl oz) can coconut milk
50 g (1¾ oz) spinach, chopped
1 tablespoon chopped coriander (cilantro)
salt and pepper
Greek yoghurt, to serve

Heat oil in a large saucepan over medium heat and cook onion and ginger for 3 minutes, or until softened. Stir in spices and, after 2 minutes, add lentils, 400 ml (13½ fl oz) boiling water and coconut milk. Bring to the boil, then simmer over low heat for 25 minutes. Add spinach and stir. Season to taste, sprinkle with coriander and serve with Greek yoghurt. Store rest of dahl in fridge for another day or freeze for later.

Dinner

CREAMY MUSHROOM & TALEGGIO POLENTA

SERVES: 1 + ENOUGH FOR CHUNKY POLENTA (PAGE 84)
PREPARATION: 5 MINUTES
COOK: 12 MINUTES

2 tablespoons extra virgin olive oil
1 garlic clove, thinly sliced
1 red onion, sliced
150 g (5½ oz) mixed mushrooms, sliced
1 tablespoon chopped parsley
125 g (4½ oz) instant polenta
30 g (1 oz) butter
50 g (1¾ oz) Taleggio cheese, sliced
salt and pepper

Heat oil in a frying pan over medium heat and fry garlic and onion for 1 minute. Add mushrooms and cook for 5 minutes. Remove from heat and add parsley. Meanwhile, bring 500 ml (2 cups) water to the boil in a large saucepan. Pour in polenta, stirring constantly for 5 minutes, or until it leaves side of pan but it is still runny. Remove from heat, add butter and season to taste. Divide mixture in half. Spread one half on a tray and store in fridge for another day. Top other half with Taleggio slices and grill until melting. Add mushrooms and serve immediately.

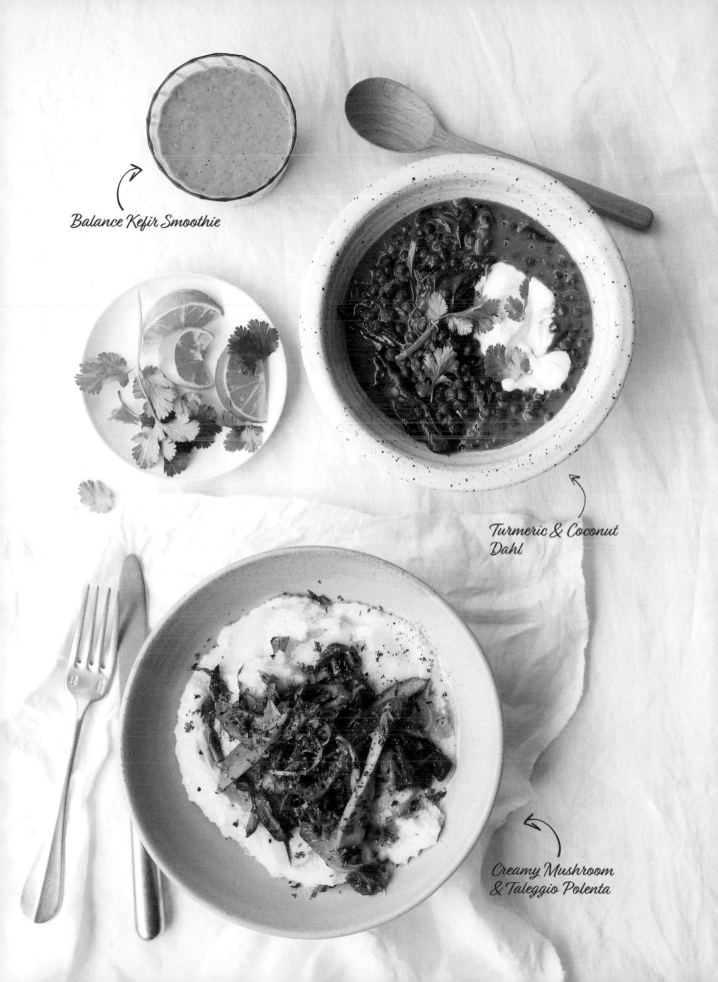

Balance Kefir Smoothie

Turmeric & Coconut
Dahl

Creamy Mushroom
& Taleggio Polenta

Tuesday

Cabbage not only has impressive health benefits, but is also cost effective and tastes delicious when caramelised and paired with the protein-rich lentils.

Breakfast

DIY GRANOLA WITH YOGHURT & FRUIT

SERVES: 1
PREPARATION: 2 MINUTES
COOK: 0 MINUTES

100 g (3½ oz) live yoghurt (page 66)
45 g (1½ oz) Granola (page 72)
100 g (3½ oz) mixed fresh fruit, sliced

Spoon half of yoghurt into base of a bowl. Add half quantity of granola and fruit. Repeat layers.

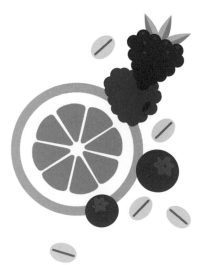

Lunch

FENNEL, GRAPEFRUIT & POPPY SEED SALAD WITH SALMON

SERVES: 1
PREPARATION: 5 MINUTES
COOK: 15 MINUTES

150 g (5½ oz) salmon fillet, skin on
30 g (1 oz) live yoghurt (page 66)
1 tablespoon extra virgin olive oil
½ teaspoon poppy seeds
1 grapefruit, cut into segments
½ fennel bulb, thinly sliced
1 teaspoon chopped chives
salt and pepper

Preheat oven to 190°C (375°F). Lay salmon, skin-side down, on a baking tray, season with salt and pepper and bake for 15 minutes, or until cooked. Cool, then flake into large chunks and set aside. Meanwhile, mix yoghurt, oil and poppy seeds together in a small bowl, then season with salt and pepper. Mix grapefruit with fennel and half the dressing, toss and arrange on a plate. Arrange salmon on top, drizzle with remaining dressing and sprinkle with chives.

Dinner

CARAMELISED ROAST CABBAGE WITH LENTILS

SERVES: 1
PREPARATION: 5 MINUTES
COOK: 35 MINUTES

4 tablespoons extra virgin olive oil
½ small red onion, chopped
80 g (2¾ oz) brown or green lentils
50 g (1¾ oz) tomatoes, chopped
1 tablespoon balsamic vinegar
2 teaspoons honey
½ small winter cabbage, halved
1 teaspoon chopped parsley
salt and pepper

Heat 1 tablespoon oil in a large saucepan over medium heat and cook onion for 3 minutes, or until softened. Add lentils, tomatoes and 150 ml (5 fl oz) hot water, bring to the boil, then simmer for 30 minutes. Season to taste. Meanwhile, combine 2 tablespoons oil, the vinegar and honey in a small bowl. Brush cabbage wedges with dressing and season with salt and pepper. Heat remaining oil in a frying pan and cook cabbage on both sides for 15 minutes, or until edges are golden brown, brushing frequently with dressing. Spoon lentils onto a plate, add cabbage wedges and sprinkle with parsley.

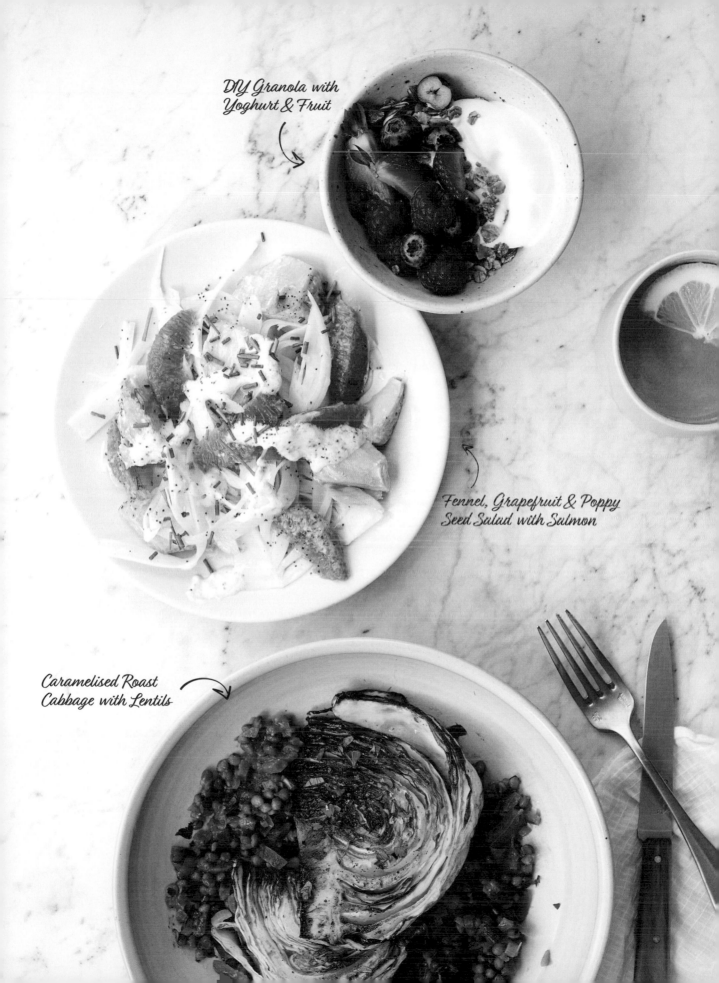

DIY Granola with
Yoghurt & Fruit

Fennel, Grapefruit & Poppy
Seed Salad with Salmon

Caramelised Roast
Cabbage with Lentils

Wednesday

A day full of fermented foods, adding depth to your diet and the health benefits that come from live microbes, which thrive in food such as kimchi, tempeh and yoghurt.

Breakfast

SMASHED EGG ON SOURDOUGH TOAST WITH KIMCHI

SERVES: 1
PREPARATION: 1 MINUTE
COOK: 3 MINUTES

2 large eggs
1 tablespoon full-fat milk
10 g (¼ oz) butter
1 slice sourdough bread, toasted
2 tablespoons kimchi
salt and pepper

Whisk eggs and milk together in a small bowl, then season with salt and pepper. Heat a small frying pan for 1 minute, then add butter and let it melt. Pour in eggs and leave for 20 seconds, then stir with a wooden spoon, mixing and folding until eggs are softly set. Arrange on toast and add kimchi.

Lunch

CHUNKY POLENTA & AVOCADO SALAD WITH TEMPEH

SERVES: 1
PREPARATION: 5 MINUTES
COOK: 10 MINUTES

½ quantity polenta (from Monday)
3 tablespoons extra virgin olive oil
50 g (1¾ oz) tempeh, cut into cubes
1 small avocado, thinly sliced
50 g (1¾ oz) baby rocket (arugula)
50 g (1¾ oz) watercress
1 tablespoon balsamic vinegar
salt

Remove polenta from fridge and put it onto a clean surface. Using a sharp knife, cut into 2 x 10 cm (¾ x 4 in) batons. Heat 1 tablespoon oil in a non-stick frying pan over medium heat and cook batons for 5 minutes, or until crisp and golden. Set aside. In same pan, heat 1 tablespoon oil, add tempeh and cook for 5 minutes, or until brown on both sides. Put avocado, rocket and watercress in a bowl, season with salt, remaining oil and vinegar, then arrange on a plate and top with polenta and tempeh. Serve.

Dinner

CHICKPEA & SAFFRON SOUP WITH LIVE YOGHURT

SERVES: 2
PREPARATION: 5 MINUTES
COOK: 10 MINUTES

1 tablespoon extra virgin olive oil
1 small red onion, finely chopped
240 g (8½ oz) canned chickpeas (garbanzo beans), drained and rinsed
300 ml (10 fl oz) vegetable stock
pinch of saffron threads
50 g (1¾ oz) live yoghurt (page 66)
1 teaspoon paprika (optional)
1 tablespoon coriander (cilantro)

Heat oil in a large saucepan over medium heat and cook onion for 3 minutes, or until softened. Stir in chickpeas and stock, bring to a simmer and cook for a few minutes. Purée 80 g (2¾ oz) of chickpeas with 200–250 ml (7–8½ fl oz) stock, then put into a bowl and whisk in saffron and yoghurt. Add a few tablespoons of broth to loosen up mixture if necessary. Whisk mixture back into soup, stirring and cooking for another 5 minutes. Ladle into a bowl and sprinkle with paprika, if liked, and coriander. Store rest of soup in fridge for another day.

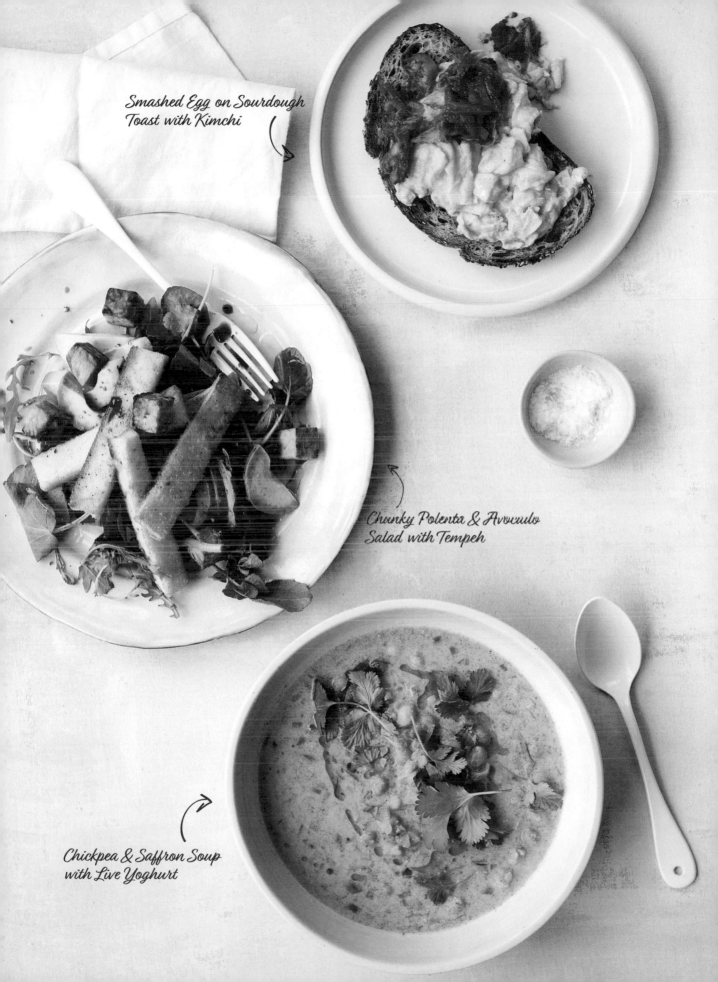

Smashed Egg on Sourdough Toast with Kimchi

Chunky Polenta & Avocado Salad with Tempeh

Chickpea & Saffron Soup with Live Yoghurt

Thursday

Cashew butter is full of monounsaturated fatty acids, healthy protein and vitamins, but try to opt for an unsweetened unsalted variety when buying.

Breakfast

STRAWBERRIES & 'CASHEW' CREAM

SERVES: 1
PREPARATION: 5 MINUTES
COOK: 0 MINUTES

45 g (1½ oz) cashew nut butter
15 g (½ oz) honey
pinch of salt
150 g (1 cup) strawberries, quartered
1 teaspoon chopped toasted nuts

Stir cashew butter, honey and salt together, adding a few tablespoons water until sauce becomes a thick consistency. Put into a serving bowl, arrange strawberries on top, then sprinkle with toasted nuts.

Lunch

HEIRLOOM TOMATO, BEAN & FETA SALAD

SERVES: 1
PREPARATION: 5 MINUTES
COOK: 0 MINUTES

150 g (5½ oz) heirloom tomatoes, sliced
50 g (1¾ oz) canned borlotti (cranberry) beans, drained and rinsed
1 tablespoon extra virgin olive oil
50 g (1¾ oz) feta, crumbled
1 tablespoon basil leaves
salt and pepper

Arrange tomatoes on a plate and season with salt. In a small bowl, season beans with a drizzle of oil, salt and pepper. Arrange beans over tomatoes, then scatter over feta and basil.

Dinner

PAPPARDELLE WITH CAVOLO NERO & PARMESAN

SERVES: 1
PREPARATION: 5 MINUTES
COOK: 10 MINUTES

80 g (2¾ oz) pappardelle pasta
60 g (2 oz) cavolo nero, tough ribs removed
2 tablespoons extra virgin olive oil
1 garlic clove, chopped
¼ teaspoon chilli flakes
25 g (1 oz) parmesan, grated
1 tablespoon mixed toasted nuts
salt and pepper

Bring 1 litre (4 cups) water to the boil in a large saucepan. Add salt and cook pasta according to packet instructions until al dente. Meanwhile, chop cavolo nero roughly and blanch it in another saucepan of boiling water for 5 minutes. Drain well. Heat oil in a frying pan and fry garlic and chilli flakes for 1 minute. Add cavolo nero, season well and cook for another 2 minutes. Drain pasta, reserving 1 tablespoon cooking water. Add pasta to frying pan and mix together thoroughly with parmesan and reserved cooking water for 1 minute. Sprinkle with toasted nuts.

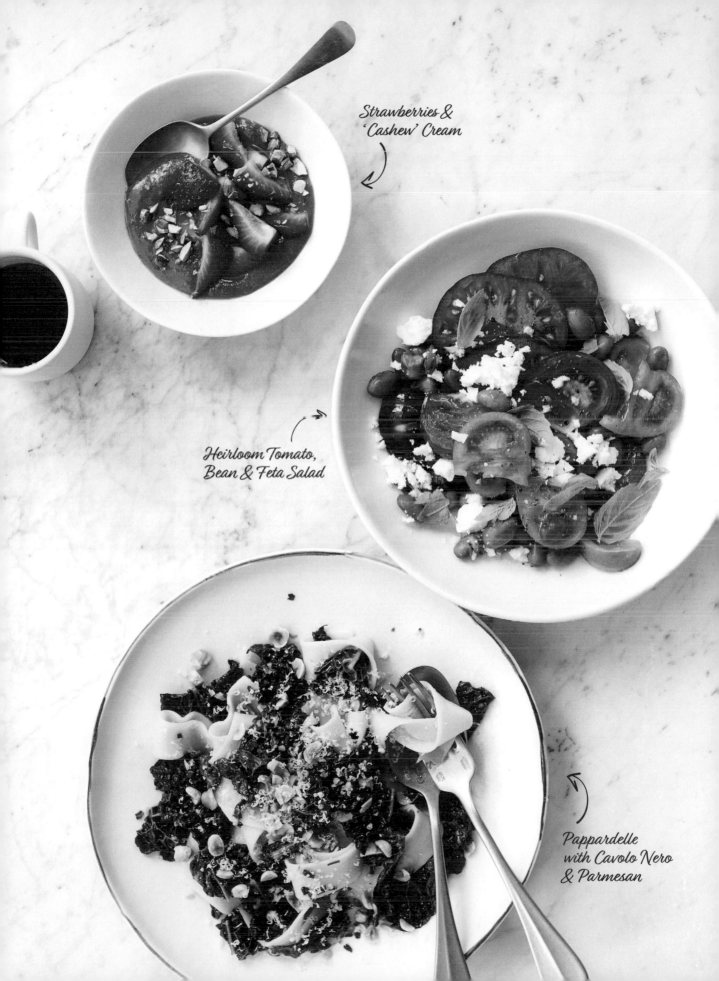

Strawberries &
'Cashew' Cream

Heirloom Tomato,
Bean & Feta Salad

Pappardelle
with Cavolo Nero
& Parmesan

Friday

Roasted harissa carrots is a recipe that should be made when carrots are fresh and young at the peak of the season. This recipe is easy to make and can be used as a side dish to many other dishes.

Breakfast

MIXED MELON & AVOCADO SALAD WITH GINGER-HONEY DRESSING

SERVES: 1
PREPARATION: 5 MINUTES
COOK: 0 MINUTES

2 teaspoons grated ginger
40 g (1½ oz) honey
2 tablespoons lime juice
3 tablespoons extra virgin olive oil
150 g (5½ oz) mixed melon, cut into 2.5 cm (1 in) wedges
½ avocado, cut into 2.5 cm (1 in) wedges
30 g (1 oz) grapes, cut lengthways
salt and pepper

Pulse ginger, honey and lime juice in a food processor to combine. While processor is running, slowly add oil to emulsify dressing. Season to taste. Put melon, avocado and grapes into a bowl, drizzle with dressing and toss to coat.

Lunch

ROASTED HARISSA CARROTS WITH LIVE LABNEH

SERVES: 1
PREPARATION: 5 MINUTES
COOK: 30 MINUTES

1 tablespoon harissa paste, plus extra to serve
1 tablespoon maple syrup
1 tablespoon extra virgin olive oil
1 teaspoon lemon juice
8 small carrots
100 g (3½ oz) labneh
2 tablespoons mixed toasted nuts
salt

Preheat oven to 190°C (375°F). In a small bowl, mix harissa, maple syrup, oil and lemon juice together, then season with salt. Set aside. Peel carrots, leaving 5 cm (2 in) of green top. Add carrots to a baking dish and drizzle with harissa sauce. Toss to coat and add 2 tablespoons water. Roast carrots for 30 minutes, or until soft, adding a splash of water if getting dry. Serve carrots with labneh and sprinkled with toasted nuts on top and a dash of harissa.

Dinner

PAN-ROASTED CHICKEN WITH ORANGE & OLIVES

SERVES: 1
PREPARATION: 40 MINUTES
COOK: 25 MINUTES

1 orange
2 bone-in chicken thighs
1 garlic clove, sliced
1 rosemary sprig
1 tablespoon extra virgin olive oil
10 black olives, pitted
large handful of kale
1 teaspoon chopped parsley
salt and pepper

Grate zest of orange, squeeze half and cut rest into slices. Set aside. In a bowl, marinate chicken thighs with orange zest and juice, garlic, rosemary and salt and pepper for 30 minutes. Heat oil in an ovenproof frying pan over medium–high heat, add chicken and cook for 3 minutes on each side. Add orange slices, olives and kale and mix thoroughly for a few minutes. Roast in oven for 15–20 minutes until chicken is cooked through. Sprinkle with parsley and serve.

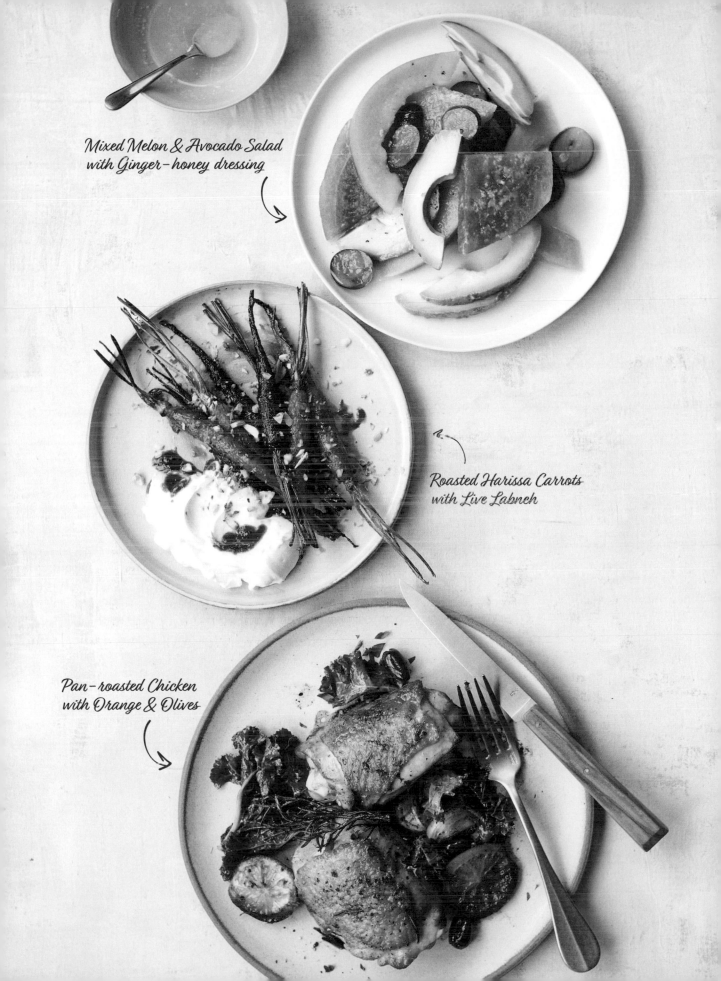

Mixed Melon & Avocado Salad
with Ginger-honey dressing

Roasted Harissa Carrots
with Live Labneh

Pan-roasted Chicken
with Orange & Olives

Saturday

A great way to add vegetables to your plate, zucchini noodles can be the star of so many dishes from pasta-style bowls to salads to stir-fries.

Breakfast

HERBY SPINACH SHAKSHUKA

SERVES: 1
PREPARATION: 5 MINUTES
COOK: 10 MINUTES

1 tablespoon extra virgin olive oil
½ garlic clove, crushed
20 g (¾ oz) mixed herbs (basil, parsley, mint)
100 g (3½ oz) spinach, roughly chopped
1 teaspoon ground turmeric
1 tablespoon lime juice
2 eggs
salt and pepper
sourdough bread (toasted) and lime wedge, to serve

Heat oil in a frying pan over medium heat and fry garlic for 1 minute, then add herbs and cook, stirring for about 5 minutes. Add spinach and mix to incorporate herbs. Add turmeric and season with salt and pepper. Add 50 ml (1¾ fl oz) water and cook until nearly evaporated, then add lime juice and mix. Make 2 small wells in spinach and crack an egg into each. Cover with a lid and cook for 3–5 minutes until eggs are set, then serve with toast and lime wedge.

Lunch

STUFFED TOMATOES

SERVES: 1
PREPARATION: 5 MINUTES
COOK: 10 MINUTES

2 tomatoes
50 g (1¾ oz) cooked brown rice
30 g (1 oz) feta, crumbled
1 teaspoon chopped mint
1 teaspoon chopped parsley
1 tablespoon extra virgin olive oil
pepper
baby salad leaves, to serve (optional)

Preheat oven to 180°C (350°F). Cut tops off tomatoes and remove flesh. Discard seeds, chop flesh and set aside with tops. Season tomatoes and put, cut-side down, on a baking tray. In a small bowl, mix tomato flesh with rice, feta and herbs and season with pepper. Divide mixture between tomatoes, drizzle with oil, cover with tomato tops and bake for 10 minutes. Serve with salad leaves, if desired.

Dinner

ZUCCHINI NOODLES WITH RICOTTA & BASIL

SERVES: 1
PREPARATION: 5 MINUTES
COOK: 2 MINUTES

2 zucchini (courgettes), 1 yellow and 1 green
1 tablespoon extra virgin olive oil
½ garlic clove, sliced
100 g (3½ oz) ricotta
1 teaspoon grated lemon zest
1 tablespoon lemon juice
1 tablespoon chopped basil
1 teaspoon toasted pumpkin seeds

Using a julienne peeler, cut zucchini into thin noodles. Heat oil in a non-stick frying pan over medium heat and fry garlic for 1 minute. Add zucchini noodles and toss to coat. Remove from heat and arrange them on a plate. Top with ricotta, grated lemon zest and juice, and basil. Sprinkle with pumpkin seeds and serve.

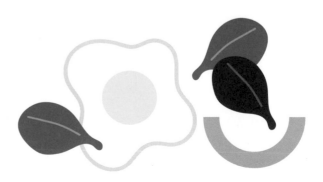

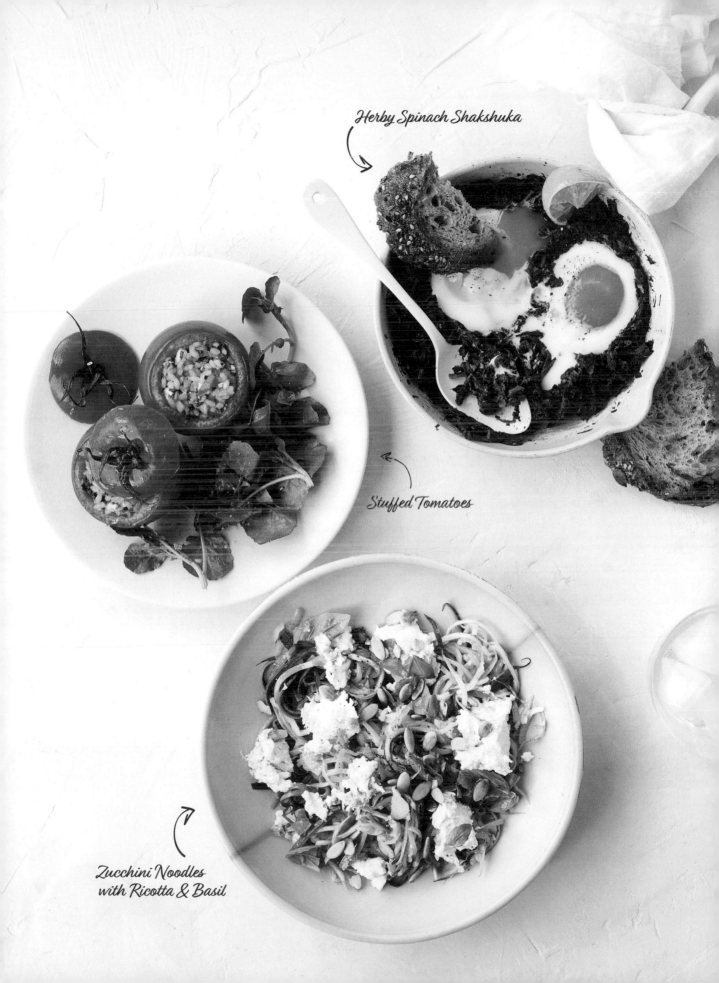

Herby Spinach Shakshuka

Stuffed Tomatoes

Zucchini Noodles
with Ricotta & Basil

Sunday

The left-over pancakes for breakfast and the stew for dinner can be stored in the fridge for up to two days. Instead of spelt in the stew, use wheat berries.

Breakfast

RYE PANCAKES WITH BLUEBERRIES & GREEK YOGHURT

SERVES: 2 / MAKES: 4
PREPARATION: 5 MINUTES
COOK: 10 MINUTES

90 g (3 oz) rye flour
85 g (3 oz) wholemeal (whole-wheat) flour
2 teaspoons baking powder
1 large egg, lightly whisked
3 tablespoons maple syrup
150 g (5½ oz) Greek yoghurt
15 g (½ oz) butter
150 g (1 cup) blueberries
salt

Whisk flours, baking powder and a pinch of salt together in a bowl. In another bowl, mix egg with 1 tablespoon maple syrup and 100 g (3½ oz) yoghurt. Add to dry ingredients and mix until just combined. Heat a frying pan over medium heat, add half the butter and let it melt. Ladle 50 g (1¾ oz) batter into pan, sprinkle with some blueberries and cook for 2 minutes. When bottom has set, flip using a palette knife and cook for another 1 minute. Repeat until all batter is used. Serve with remaining blueberries, yoghurt and syrup.

Lunch

PAN-ROASTED MACKEREL WITH FENNEL & CAPERS

SERVES: 1
PREPARATION: 10 MINUTES
COOK: 13 MINUTES

1 teaspoon salted capers
1 tablespoon extra virgin olive oil
1 small fennel bulb, cut into wedges
2 mackerel fillets or fish of choice
juice of ½ lemon
salt and pepper
lemon wedge, to serve

Soak capers for 5 minutes, then rinse and repeat twice more. Drain. Heat oil in a non-stick frying pan over medium heat and cook fennel for 3 minutes. Add capers and cook for another 2 minutes, then set aside. Season fish with salt and pepper, add to pan and cook for 3 minutes each side. Add fennel mixture and lemon juice and cook for another 2 minutes. Serve with lemon wedge.

Dinner

SPELT & BEAN STEW

SERVES: 2
PREPARATION: 5 MINUTES
COOK: 40 MINUTES

2 tablespoons extra virgin olive oil, plus extra for drizzling
50 g (1¾ oz) soffritto (red onion, celery, carrot), chopped
5 cherry tomatoes, halved
100 g (3½ oz) spelt
300 ml (10 fl oz) vegetable stock
50 g (1¾ oz) spinach, roughly chopped
100 g (3½ oz) canned cannellini beans, drained and rinsed

Heat oil in a large saucepan over medium heat and cook soffritto and tomatoes for 3 minutes. Add spelt and cook for another 3 minutes, stirring constantly. Add stock, bring to the boil, then simmer for 30 minutes, or until spelt is tender. Stir spinach and beans into soup and cook for another 5 minutes until spinach wilts. Drizzle with oil. Store rest of stew in fridge for another day.

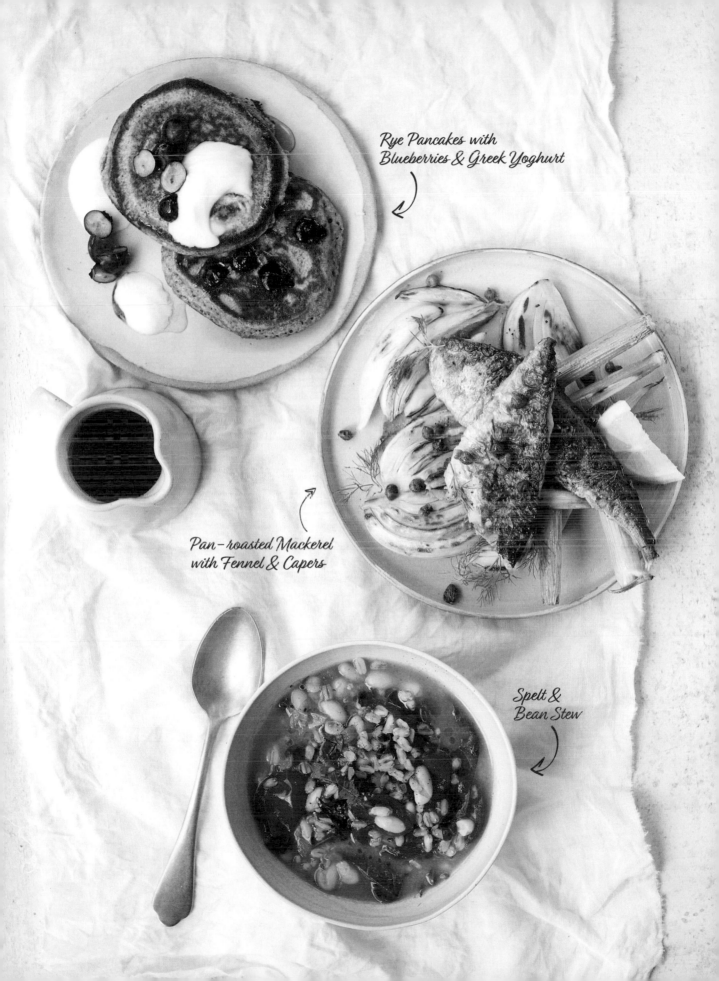

Rye Pancakes with
Blueberries & Greek Yoghurt

Pan-roasted Mackerel
with Fennel & Capers

Spelt &
Bean Stew

Vegetables

- ○ 150 g (5½ oz) butternut squash
- ○ 300 g (10½ oz) purple potatoes
- ○ 100 g (3½ oz) mixed mushrooms + 1 large flat mushroom
- ○ 20 g (¾ oz) rocket (arugula)
- ○ 60 g (2 oz) watercress
- ○ 1 large tomato
- ○ 50 g (1¾ oz) green beans
- ○ 2 yellow zucchini (courgettes)
- ○ 1 green zucchini (courgette)
- ○ 1 round purple or big black eggplant (aubergine)
- ○ 600 g (1 lb 5 oz) cherry tomatoes
- ○ 110 g (4 oz) ripe tomatoes
- ○ 80 g (2¾ oz) broccoli
- ○ 30 g (1 oz) kale leaves
- ○ 1 small cucumber
- ○ 500 g (1 lb 2 oz) cauliflower
- ○ 50 g (1¾ oz) yellow bell pepper (capsicum)
- ○ 1 avocado
- ○ 1½ small red onions
- ○ 1 French shallot
- ○ 2½ garlic cloves
- ○ 1 tsp grated fresh ginger
- ○ 4 tbsp soffritto (onion, carrot, celery)
- ○ 3 spring (green) onions
- ○ 2½ tbsp parsley
- ○ 80 g (2¾ oz) basil leaves
- ○ 2½ tbsp mint leaves
- ○ ½ lemongrass stalk
- ○ 1½ tsp oregano
- ○ 20 g (¾ oz) mixed sprouts

Fruit

- ○ 2 bananas
- ○ ½ apple
- ○ 2 dried apricots
- ○ 80 g (½ cup) blueberries
- ○ 1 tbsp berries
- ○ 100 ml (3½ fl oz) organic apple juice
- ○ 50 g (1¾ oz) mixed fresh fruit
- ○ 1 pink grapefruit
- ○ 1 orange
- ○ 2 tbsp lime juice
- ○ 3 tbsp lemon juice + grated zest 1 lemon + lemon wedge
- ○ 1 peach
- ○ 25 g (1 oz) pomegranate seeds

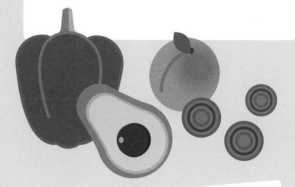

Fridge Products

- ○ 150 g (5½ oz) beef rump steak
- ○ 2 lamb chops
- ○ 100 g (3½ oz) frozen mixed seafood, thawed
- ○ 2 mackerel fillets
- ○ 975 ml (33 fl oz) vegetable stock
- ○ 1 tbsp pickles (gherkins) + 65 g (2¼ oz) pickled radish

In the Storecupboard

- ○ 4 slices sourdough bread + 50 g (1¾ oz) sourdough bread
- ○ 75 g (2¾ oz) paella rice
- ○ 250 g (9 oz) cannellini beans
- ○ 200 g (7 oz) canned roma (plum) tomatoes
- ○ 200 g (7 oz) canned chopped tomatoes
- ○ 50 g (1¾ oz) chickpeas (garbanzo beans)
- ○ 50 g (1¾ oz) millet
- ○ 80 g (2¾ oz) pearl barley
- ○ 50 g (1¾ oz) freekeh
- ○ 20 g (¾ oz) rolled (porridge) oats
- ○ 20 g (¾ oz) barley flakes
- ○ 20 g (¾ oz) rye flakes
- ○ 130 g (4½ oz) almond flour
- ○ 40 g (1½ oz) oat flour
- ○ 60 g (2 oz) plain (all-purpose) flour
- ○ 90 g (3 oz) wholemeal (whole-wheat) flour
- ○ 125 g (4½ oz) besan (chickpea flour)
- ○ 50 g (1¾ oz) wholemeal couscous
- ○ 1 tablespoon white wine
- ○ 115 ml (4 fl oz) maple syrup
- ○ 50 g (1¾ oz) triple nut butter
- ○ 1 tbsp toasted nuts
- ○ 2½ tbsp pine nuts
- ○ extra virgin olive oil
- ○ balsamic vinegar
- ○ white wine vinegar
- ○ ground turmeric
- ○ chilli flakes
- ○ sumac

- ○ saffron
- ○ ground cinnamon
- ○ baking powder and baking soda
- ○ harissa spice
- ○ honey

Eggs & Dairy Products

- ○ 2 tbsp butter
- ○ 100 g (3½ oz) halloumi
- ○ 65 g (2¼ oz) parmesan
- ○ 2 tbsp cream
- ○ 50 g (1¾ oz) mozzarella
- ○ 150 g (5½ oz) burrata
- ○ 50 g (1¾ oz) feta
- ○ 340 ml (1⅓ cups) kefir milk
- ○ 2 tbsp Greek yoghurt
- ○ 145 g (5 oz) live yoghurt
- ○ 4 eggs + 1 egg yolk

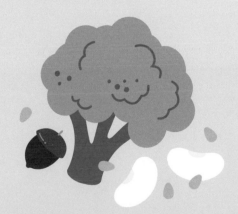

Monday

Wholegrain freekeh contains more fibre and protein than standard wheat and it is a source of calcium, potassium, iron and zinc. It is a good addition to soups and salads.

Breakfast

TRIPLE NUT BUTTER TOAST WITH BANANA

SERVES: 1
PREPARATION: 5 MINUTES
COOK: 2 MINUTES

1 slice sourdough bread
50 g (1¾ oz) triple nut butter
   (page 70)
1 banana, sliced

Toast bread, spread with nut butter and arrange banana slices over.

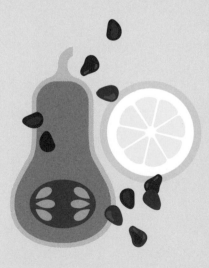

Lunch

ROAST SQUASH, HALLOUMI & FREEKEH WARM SALAD

SERVES: 1
PREPARATION: 5 MINUTES
COOK: 25 MINUTES

150 g (5½ oz) butternut squash,
   peeled and cut into 2–3 cm
   (¾–1¼ in) chunks
2 tablespoons extra virgin olive oil
1 teaspoon harissa spice
50 g (1¾ oz) freekeh
50 g (1¾ oz) halloumi, sliced
1 tablespoon lemon juice
25 g (1 oz) pomegranate seeds
salt and pepper

Preheat oven to 180°C (350°F). Put squash into a roasting dish, toss with oil, harissa and season to taste. Roast for 20 minutes, or until squash is golden and softened, turning them over after 10 minutes. Meanwhile bring 400 ml (13½ fl oz) water to the boil in a medium saucepan. Add freekeh and simmer for 20 minutes, or until tender. Stir freekeh into roasting dish and roast for another 2 minutes. Heat a frying pan over high heat and fry halloumi for 1–2 minutes on each side until golden. Transfer squash and freekeh mix to a plate, add lemon juice and mix. Arrange halloumi on top and sprinkle over pomegranate seeds.

Dinner

GNOCCHI WITH MUSHROOM RAGOUT

SERVES: 2
PREPARATION: 5 MINUTES
COOK: 30 MINUTES

300 g (10½ oz) purple potatoes,
   peeled and halved
60 g (2 oz) plain (all-purpose) flour
1 egg yolk, whisked
1 tablespoon extra virgin olive oil
½ garlic clove, chopped
100 g (3½ oz) mixed mushrooms,
   sliced
1 tablespoon grated parmesan
1 teaspoon chopped parsley
salt

Boil potatoes in a pan of water until tender. Drain, cool and mash in a bowl. Add flour, salt and egg yolk and mix well. Transfer to a lightly floured work surface and knead to a dough. Divide dough into pieces and roll each piece into a long sausage, 2 cm (¾ in) in diameter. Cut sausage into 1.5–2 cm (½–¾ in) chunks, then press down gently on each chunk with a fork. Leave on a plate, spaced apart. Heat oil in a frying pan and fry garlic and mushrooms for 5 minutes. Bring 500 ml (2 cups) salted water to the boil and cook gnocchi until they float on surface. Using a slotted spoon, transfer them to frying pan and fry for 2 minutes with parmesan and parsley. Serve. Store rest in fridge for another day.

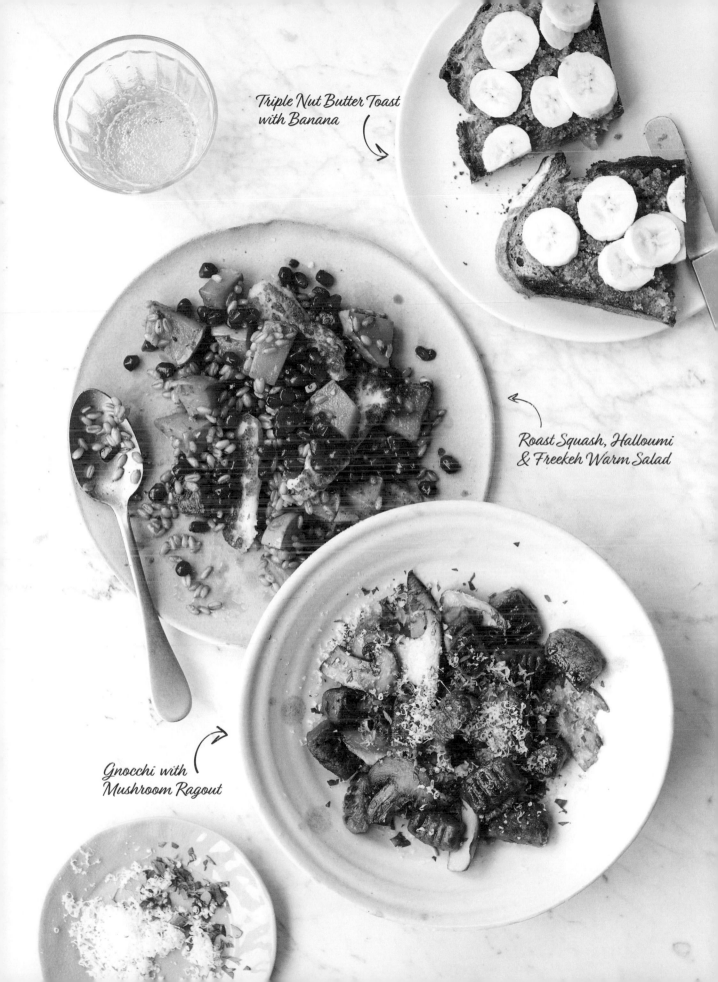

*Triple Nut Butter Toast
with Banana*

*Roast Squash, Halloumi
& Freekeh Warm Salad*

*Gnocchi with
Mushroom Ragout*

Tuesday

Created to get people to eat more fruit, Bircher muesli is great for a quick breakfast, simple and delicious with the smoothness of the oats and the crunchiness of the apple. You can use an unpeeled pear instead.

Breakfast

BIRCHER MUESLI

SERVES: 1
PREPARATION: 5 MINUTES
SOAK: OVERNIGHT

½ apple, unpeeled and coarsely grated
20 g (¾ oz) rolled (porridge) oats
20 g (¾ oz) barley flakes
20 g (¾ oz) rye flakes
2 dried apricots, chopped
100 ml (3½ fl oz) organic apple juice
1 tablespoon berries
1 tablespoon chopped toasted nuts

Put apple, oats, barley and rye flakes, apricots and apple juice into a bowl and stir well. Cover bowl and leave to soak overnight in fridge. Next morning, stir muesli, then top with berries and nuts.

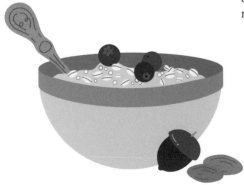

Lunch

CHARGRILLED STEAK & PICKLE OPEN SANDWICH

SERVES: 1
PREPARATION: 5 MINUTES
COOK: 10 MINUTES

150 g (5½ oz) beef rump steak
1 large flat mushroom
2 tablespoons extra virgin olive oil
1 large slice sourdough bread
20 g (¾ oz) rocket (arugula)
1 tablespoon pickled radish (page 74)
1 tablespoon pickles (gherkins)
salt and pepper

Preheat a chargrill pan over medium heat. Drizzle steak and mushroom with 1 tablespoon oil, season and cook for 4 minutes on each side until cooked to your preference. Let steak rest 5 minutes before slicing. Brush bread with remaining oil and cook in pan for 30 seconds on each side. Top with mushroom, rocket, steak, radish and pickles.

Dinner

PROVENÇAL PISTOU SOUP

SERVES: 2
PREPARATION: 5 MINUTES
COOK: 20 MINUTES

80 ml (⅓ cup) extra virgin olive oil
2 tablespoons soffritto (finely chopped onion, carrot, celery)
1 large tomato, peeled and chopped
50 g (1¾ oz) green beans, sliced into 5 cm (2 in) pieces
1 yellow zucchini (courgette), diced
200 g (7 oz) canned cannellini beans, drained and rinsed
½ garlic clove
50 g (1¾ oz) basil leaves
20 g (¾ oz) parmesan, grated
salt and pepper

Heat 2 tablespoons oil in a large saucepan over medium heat and cook soffritto for 3 minutes. Add tomato, cook for a few minutes, then stir in green beans and zucchini and cook for 5 minutes, stirring. Add cannellini beans and 250 ml (1 cup) water or just enough to cover vegetables. Bring to the boil, then simmer for 10 minutes. Meanwhile, add garlic, basil, parmesan, pinch of salt and remaining 60 ml (¼ cup) oil to a blender and blend until basil is finely chopped. Season soup to taste, ladle into a bowl and top with a dollop of pistou. Store both in fridge for another day.

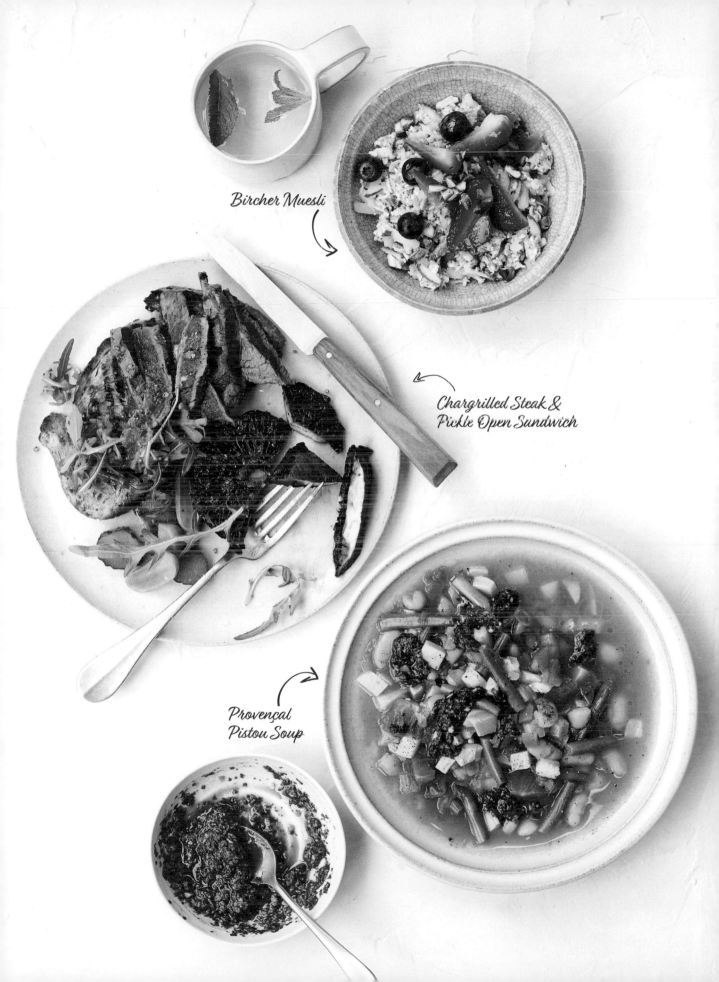

Bircher Muesli

*Chargrilled Steak &
Pickle Open Sandwich*

*Provençal
Pistou Soup*

Wednesday

A source of fibre and low in fat and sugar, eggplants are full of vitamins and minerals. Grilling them will make this classic bake even healthier.

Breakfast

ONE-POT EGG WITH SPRING ONION

SERVES: 1
PREPARATION: 5 MINUTES
COOK: 12 MINUTES

2 tablespoons cream
1 teaspoon chopped parsley
¼ teaspoon chilli flakes
2 spring (green) onions, roughly chopped
1 egg
¼ teaspoon sumac
salt and pepper
1 slice sourdough bread, toasted

Preheat oven to 170°C (340°F). Butter a ramekin dish and add 1 tablespoon cream, then add parsley, chilli flakes and half spring onion. Make an indent in mix and crack in egg. Add another tablespoon cream, season with salt and pepper and put ramekin into a small roasting dish half-filled with hot water. Bake for 12 minutes, then sprinkle remaining spring onions and sumac on top. Serve with toast.

Lunch

EGGPLANT PARMIGIANA

SERVES: 2
PREPARATION: 20 MINUTES
COOK: 30 MINUTES

1 round purple or big black eggplant (aubergine), cut into 5 mm (¼ in) slices
1 tablespoon extra virgin olive oil
½ small red onion, chopped
200 g (7 oz) can roma (plum) tomatoes, mashed
15 g (½ oz) basil leaves
50 g (1¾ oz) mozzarella, drained and sliced
1 tablespoon grated parmesan
salt

Put eggplant into a colander and sprinkle salt between layers. Put a plate on top, then a weight over plate and leave in sink for 15 minutes. Preheat oven to 180°C (350°F). Heat oil in a large saucepan over medium heat and cook onion for 3 minutes. Add tomatoes, splash of water and 2 basil leaves. Season with salt and cook for 15 minutes. Rinse eggplant and pat dry. Heat a griddle pan and grill eggplant for 8 minutes on both sides. Spread a spoonful of tomato sauce in a small ovenproof dish and alternate with layers of eggplant, sauce, mozzarella, parmesan and basil until all ingredients are used. Bake in oven for 25 minutes. Rest 30 minutes, then serve. Store rest in fridge for another day.

Dinner

SEAFOOD PAELLA

SERVES: 1
PREPARATION: 5 MINUTES
COOK: 25 MINUTES

½ tablespoon extra virgin olive oil
¼ small red onion, chopped
75 g (2¾ oz) paella rice
1 tablespoon white wine
100 g (3½ oz) can chopped tomatoes
225 ml (7½ fl oz) vegetable stock
½ large pinch of saffron
100 g (3½ oz) frozen mixed seafood, thawed and sliced
½ tablespoon chopped parsley
salt and pepper

Heat oil in a large frying pan over medium heat and fry onion for 3 minutes. Add rice and stir for 1 minute, splash in wine and once evaporated, add tomatoes, stock and saffron. Season and cook for 15 minutes, stirring occasionally. Add seafood, mix and simmer for 5 minutes, then sprinkle over parsley and serve immediately.

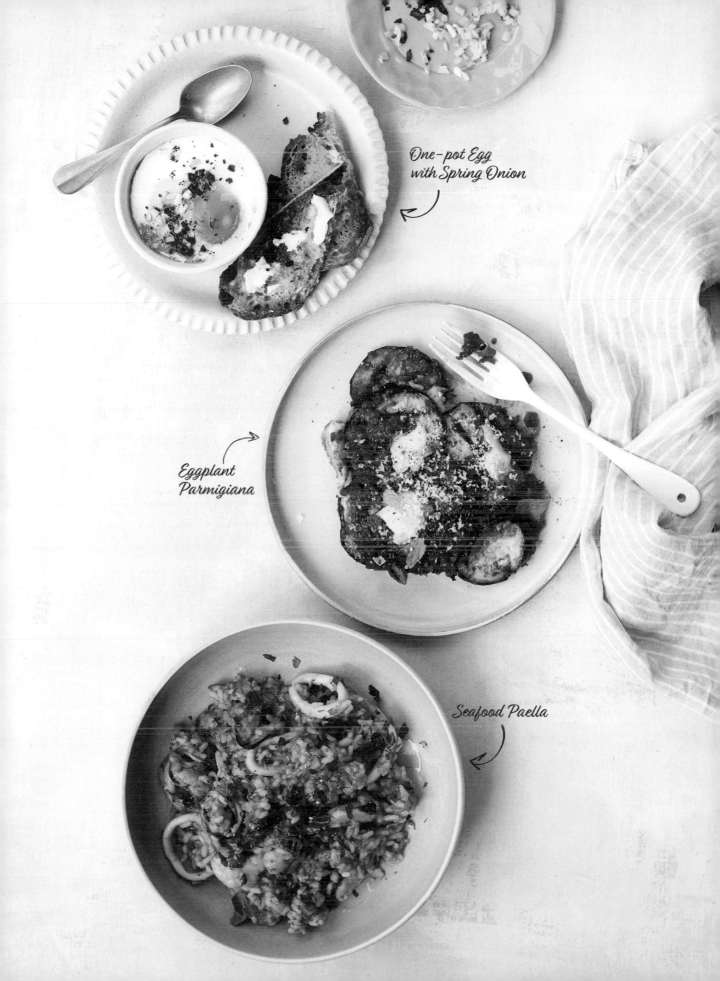

One-pot Egg
with Spring Onion

Eggplant
Parmigiana

Seafood Paella

Thursday

Even if the live probiotic culture will die when the kefir is heated, being 99 per cent lactose-free makes it a good substitute for those who are lactose intolerant. It will also make these pancakes extra fluffy.

Breakfast

ALMOND & KEFIR PANCAKES WITH FRUIT & YOGHURT

SERVES: 2 / MAKES: 4
PREPARATION: 5 MINUTES
COOK: 10 MINUTES

1 large egg, separated
70 g (2½ oz) almond flour
40 g (1½ oz) oat flour
1 teaspoon baking powder
½ teaspoon ground cinnamon
140 ml (4½ fl oz) kefir milk
butter, for frying
2 tablespoons Greek yoghurt
50 g (1¾ oz) fresh fruit

Whisk egg white in a bowl. Whisk egg yolk, flours, baking powder, cinnamon and kefir in another bowl until smooth, then fold in egg white. Heat a frying pan over medium heat, add a dollop of butter and let it melt, then pour in 1 tablespoon of batter and cook for 2–3 minutes on each side, flipping over with a spatula. Repeat until all the batter is used. Serve with yoghurt and fruit. Store rest in fridge for another day.

Lunch

BALSAMIC ZUCCHINI, FETA & PINE NUT SALAD

SERVES: 1
PREPARATION: 5 MINUTES
COOK: 0 MINUTES

1 tablespoon balsamic vinegar
1 tablespoon extra virgin olive oil
1 tablespoon lemon juice
1 green zucchini (courgette), cut lengthways into 3 mm (¼ in) slices
1 yellow zucchini (courgette), cut lengthways into 3 mm (¼ in) slices
1 tablespoon mint leaves
1 tablespoon pine nuts, toasted
50 g (1¾ oz) feta, crumbled
salt and pepper

Put vinegar into a small bowl and season with salt and pepper. Gradually whisk in oil and lemon juice. Put zucchini into a large bowl with mint and drizzle over dressing. Toss gently to combine, then sprinkle over feta, pine nuts and serve.

Dinner

BARLEY, CANNELLINI, TOMATO & WATERCRESS STEW

SERVES: 2
PREPARATION: 5 MINUTES
COOK: 35 MINUTES

80 g (2¾ oz) pearl barley
2 tablespoons extra virgin olive oil
1 French shallot, sliced
½ teaspoon chilli flakes
250 ml (1 cup) vegetable stock
50 g (1¾ oz) canned cannellini beans, drained and rinsed
2 tomatoes, chopped
60 g (2 oz) watercress
1 tablespoon grated parmesan
salt and pepper

Put barley into a medium saucepan, cover with water and cook for 20 minutes. Drain and set aside. Heat 1 tablespoon oil in another pan over medium heat and cook shallot and chilli flakes for 2 minutes. Add stock, simmer for 5 minutes, then add barley, beans and tomatoes and cook for 10 minutes. Season to taste. Blitz 30 g (1 oz) watercress with remaining oil and parmesan in a food processor until smooth. Ladle soup into a bowl, swirl in watercress salsa and top with remaining watercress. Store rest in fridge for another day.

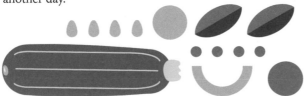

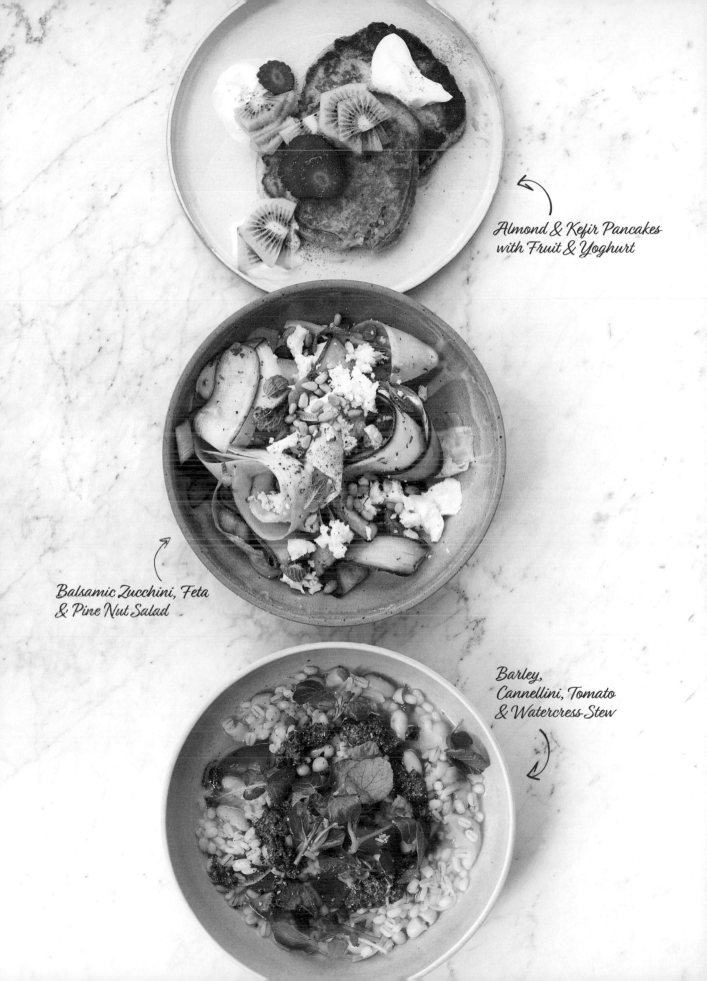

Almond & Kefir Pancakes with Fruit & Yoghurt

Balsamic Zucchini, Feta & Pine Nut Salad

Barley, Cannellini, Tomato & Watercress Stew

Friday

Kale, a very popular leafy green from the cruciferous family, is rich in nutrients. Freeze the rest of the soup for later, then defrost before reheating until piping hot.

Breakfast

CITRUS SALAD WITH LEMONGRASS, GINGER & TOASTED NUTS

SERVES: 1
PREPARATION: 5 MINUTES
COOK: 0 MINUTES

1 tablespoon lime juice
1 teaspoon grated fresh ginger
½ lemongrass stalk, thinly sliced
1 tablespoon honey
1 pink grapefruit
1 orange, peeled and sliced
    crossways
1 teaspoon pine nuts, toasted
1 teaspoon mint leaves

Combine lime juice, ginger, lemongrass and honey in a small bowl and set aside. Using a small knife, peel and remove white pith from grapefruit, then cut in between membrane to release segments. Arrange fruits on a plate, drizzle over juice mixture and sprinkle with pine nuts and mint.

Lunch

CHARRED-ROASTED BROCCOLI & HALLOUMI MILLET PILAF

SERVES: 1
PREPARATION: 5 MINUTES
COOK: 20 MINUTES

80 g (2¾ oz) broccoli, cut into small
    florets
50 g (1¾ oz) halloumi, sliced
2 tablespoons extra virgin oil
½ teaspoon chilli powder
½ teaspoon oregano
50 g (1¾ oz) millet
20 g (¾ oz) mixed sprouts
1 tablespoon lime juice
salt and pepper

Preheat oven to 200°C (400°F). Put broccoli and halloumi into a roasting tray. Drizzle with 1 tablespoon oil, add chilli and oregano, season with salt and pepper, then toss well. Bake for 15–20 minutes. Toast millet in a medium saucepan for 2 minutes. Very carefully add 100 ml (3½ fl oz) water, a pinch of salt and stir. Bring to the boil, then simmer for 15 minutes. Leave off heat for 10 minutes, then fluff with a fork. Put millet, broccoli, halloumi and sprouts onto a platter and mix together, adding remaining oil, lime juice and salt if needed.

Dinner

ROAST TOMATO & CRISPY KALE SOUP

SERVES: 2
PREPARATION: 5 MINUTES
COOK: 50 MINUTES

600 g (1 lb 5 oz) cherry tomatoes
3 tablespoons extra virgin olive oil
2 tablespoons soffritto (finely
    chopped onion, carrot, celery)
50 g (1¾ oz) canned chickpeas
    (garbanzo beans), drained
    and rinsed
250 ml (1 cup) vegetable stock
30 g (1 oz) kale leaves, stems removed
    and leaves cut into small pieces
1 tablespoon live yoghurt (page 66)
salt and pepper

Preheat oven to 200°C (400°F). Put tomatoes into a roasting tray and toss with 1 tablespoon oil. Season with salt and roast for 35 minutes. Reduce oven temperature to 160°C (320°F). Heat 1 tablespoon oil in a saucepan over medium heat and cook soffritto for 5 minutes. Add tomatoes, chickpeas and stock, then blitz with a stick blender until smooth. Coat kale with remaining oil, season, spread out over a baking tray and bake for 10 minutes, or until crisp, tossing after 5 minutes. Ladle soup into a bowl, swirl in a spoonful of yoghurt and sprinkle with crispy kale.

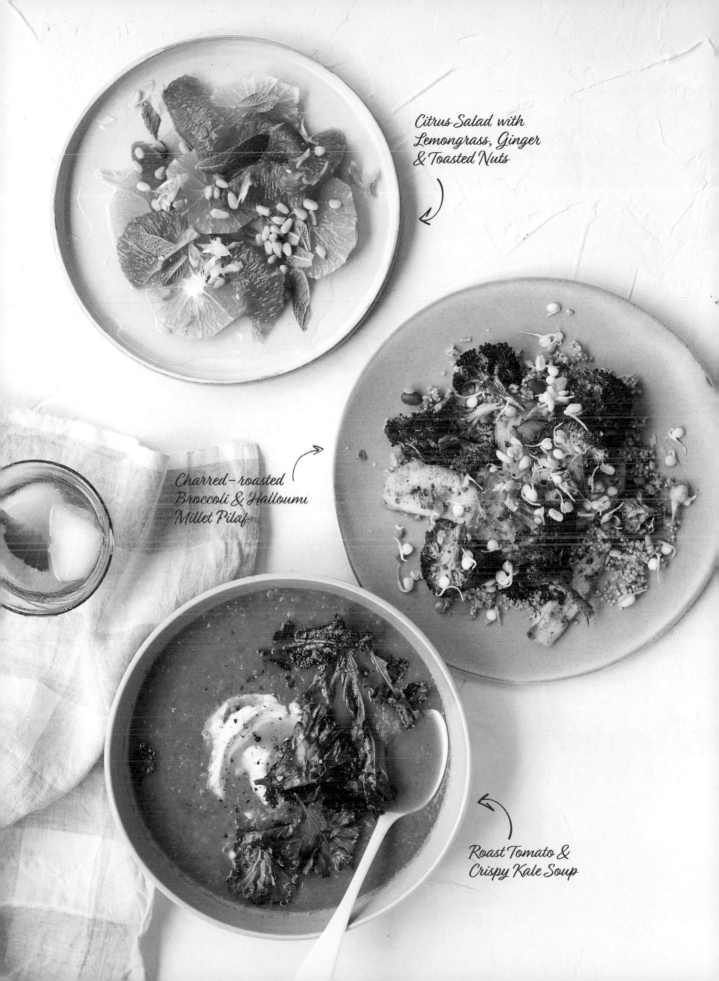

Citrus Salad with
Lemongrass, Ginger
& Toasted Nuts

Charred-roasted
Broccoli & Halloumi
Millet Pilaf

Roast Tomato &
Crispy Kale Soup

Saturday

Store the remaining muffins for breakfast either in an airtight container in the fridge for two days or freeze them for another time. If there is too much cauliflower purée for dinner then store in the fridge for three days.

Breakfast

BANANA & BLUEBERRY KEFIR MUFFINS

MAKES: 6
PREPARATION: 5 MINUTES
COOK: 25 MINUTES

90 g (3 oz) wholemeal (whole-wheat) flour
60 g (2 oz) almond flour
1 teaspoon baking powder
1 teaspoon baking soda
pinch of salt
1 tablespoon extra virgin olive oil
1 ripe banana, mashed
115 ml (4 fl oz) maple syrup
200 ml (7 fl oz) kefir milk
80 g (½ cup) blueberries

Preheat oven to 180°C (350°F). Line a 6-hole muffin tin with paper cases. Mix flours, baking powder, baking soda and salt together. In another bowl, mix oil, banana, syrup and kefir. Combine both mixtures and mix gently to just combine. Add half quantity of blueberries and mix again. Divide batter into muffin cases, top each muffin with 2 blueberries. Bake for 25 minutes, or until golden brown.

Lunch

PANZANELLA SALAD WITH TOMATOES, BURRATA & PEACH

SERVES: 1
PREPARATION: 5 MINUTES
COOK: 5 MINUTES

110 g (4 oz) ripe tomatoes, chopped into bite-sized pieces
1 tablespoon extra virgin olive oil, plus extra for drizzling
50 g (1¾ oz) sourdough bread, cut into cubes
1 peach, thinly sliced
1 tablespoon basil leaves
1 small cucumber, thinly sliced
150 g (5½ oz) burrata, torn
salt

Put tomatoes into a bowl and season with salt. Set aside. Heat 1 tablespoon oil in a frying pan, add bread cubes and toast, tossing until golden brown. Transfer tomatoes and bread to a serving bowl, add peach, basil and cucumber. Drizzle with oil and add burrata.

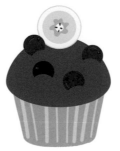

Dinner

MEDITERRANEAN MACKEREL WITH CAULIFLOWER PURÉE

SERVES: 1
PREPARATION: 5 MINUTES
COOK: 25 MINUTES

500 g (1 lb 2 oz) cauliflower, chopped
125 g (4½ oz) live yoghurt (page 66)
250 ml (1 cup) vegetable stock
1 tablespoon butter
½ garlic clove, grated
1 teaspoon white wine vinegar
1 teaspoon oregano
1 tablespoon extra virgin olive oil, plus extra to drizzle
2 mackerel fillets
salt and pepper
lemon wedge, to serve

Bring cauliflower, yoghurt and stock to the boil in a large saucepan, then simmer for 20 minutes. Drain cauliflower and reserve 2 tablespoons of cooking liquid. Blitz cauliflower and butter in a food processor, and, if necessary, the reserved liquid, until smooth. Combine garlic, vinegar, oregano and oil in a small bowl. Season. Drizzle fillets with oil and season. Cook, skin-side down first, in a frying pan for 2 minutes on each side. Put purée onto a plate, top with fish and drizzle over dressing. Serve with lemon wedge.

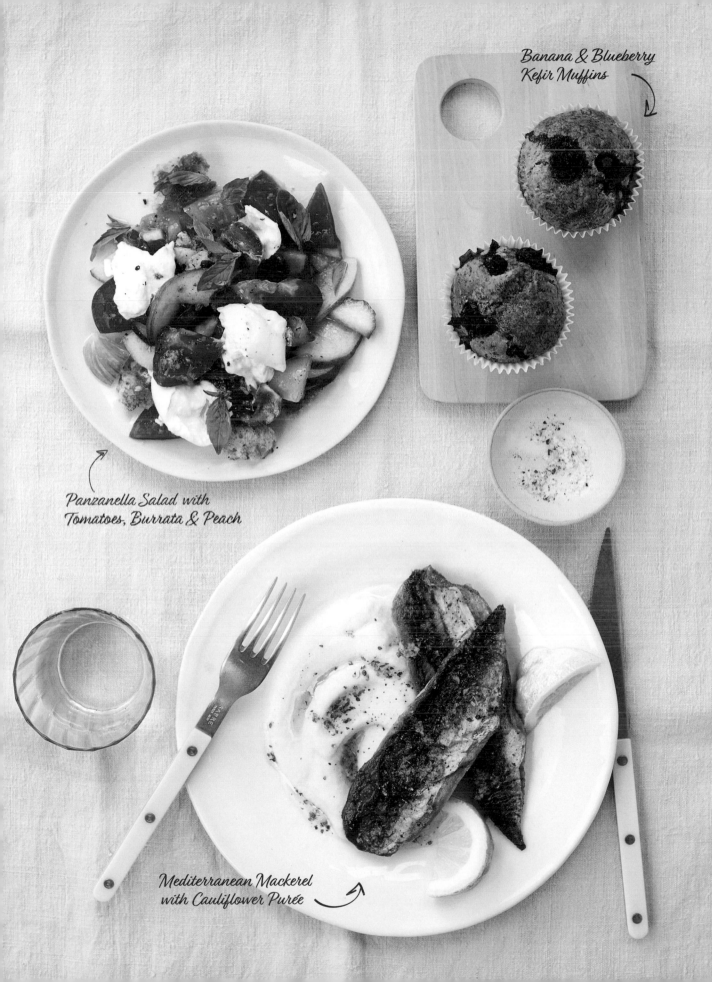

*Banana & Blueberry
Kefir Muffins*

*Panzanella Salad with
Tomatoes, Burrata & Peach*

*Mediterranean Mackerel
with Cauliflower Purée*

Sunday

Any remaining chickpea pancakes for lunch can be wrapped up and kept in the fridge for three days. Just reheat them in a pan until they are warm throughout.

Breakfast

BAKED EGGS WITH TOMATOES & BELL PEPPER

SERVES: 1
PREPARATION: 5 MINUTES
COOK: 10 MINUTES

1 tablespoon extra virgin olive oil
½ small red onion, thinly sliced
100 g (3½ oz) can chopped tomatoes
50 g (1¾ oz) yellow bell pepper
  (capsicum), sliced
2 eggs
½ teaspoon chilli flakes
1 slice sourdough bread, toasted

Heat oil in a large frying pan over medium heat and fry onion for 3 minutes. Add tomatoes, pepper and 50 ml (1¾ fl oz) water, bring to the boil, then simmer for 5 minutes. Make 2 indents and crack in eggs, then cover and cook over low heat until eggs are ready. Sprinkle with chilli flakes and serve on toast.

Lunch

CHICKPEA PANCAKES WITH AVOCADO & PICKLES

SERVES: 1
PREPARATION: 5 MINUTES
COOK: 10 MINUTES

1 teaspoon live yoghurt (page 66)
1 teaspoon lemon juice
1 avocado, roughly mashed
2 tablespoons extra virgin olive oil
1 spring (green) onion, finely chopped
¼ teaspoon ground turmeric
1 teaspoon chopped parsley
125 g (4½ oz) besan (chickpea flour)
1 teaspoon baking powder
salt and pepper
50 g (1¾ oz) pickled radish (page 74),
  to serve

Combine yoghurt, lemon juice and avocado in a bowl. Season. Heat 1 tablespoon oil in a frying pan and fry spring onion, turmeric and parsley for 3 minutes. Season and set aside. Whisk flour and baking powder together in a large bowl, then while whisking, slowly add 150 ml (5 fl oz) water to a smooth, thick but not quite pourable batter. Mix in spring onion mixture. Whisk until smooth. Heat a frying pan over medium heat and add remaining oil. Add a quarter of the batter and cook for 2 minutes on each side. Remove and keep pancake warm. Repeat with remaining batter. Serve with avocado mix and pickled radish.

Dinner

MARINATED LAMB CHOPS WITH COUSCOUS SALAD

SERVES: 1
PREPARATION: 40 MINUTES
COOK: 20 MINUTES

50 g (1¾ oz) wholemeal couscous
1 tablespoon each chopped mint
  and parsley
1 tablespoon pine nuts, toasted
grated zest and juice of 1 lemon
1 garlic clove, very finely chopped
4 tablespoons extra virgin olive oil
2 lamb chops

Cook couscous according to packet instructions, then put it into a bowl with herbs, pine nuts, half of lemon zest and juice. Set aside. Combine remaining lemon zest and juice, the parsley, garlic and oil and use to coat lamb chops on both sides. Cover and rest in fridge for 30 minutes. Heat grill to high and grill lamb chops for 5 minutes on each side, or until internal temperature is 55°C (130°F). Cover with foil and rest for 5 minutes before serving with couscous.

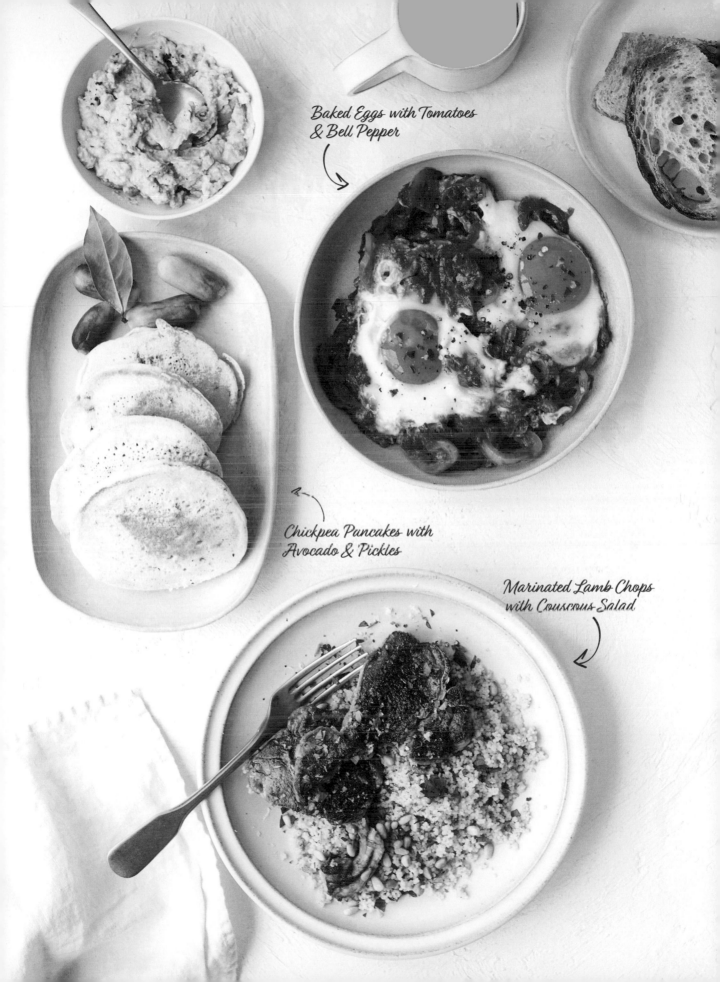

Baked Eggs with Tomatoes
& Bell Pepper

Chickpea Pancakes with
Avocado & Pickles

Marinated Lamb Chops
with Couscous Salad

Fruit

- ○ 530 g (1 lb 3 oz) fresh raspberries
- ○ 1 tbsp mixed berries
- ○ 50 g (1¾ oz) fresh or dried blueberries
- ○ 2 bananas
- ○ 1 tbsp pomegranate seeds
- ○ 2 tbsp lemon juice + 2 lemons

Eggs & Dairy Products

- ○ 1 small mozzarella ball
- ○ 30 g (1 oz) parmesan
- ○ 80 g (2¾ oz) goat's cheese
- ○ 100 g (3½ oz) feta
- ○ 50 g (1¾ oz) labneh
- ○ 45 g (1½ oz) butter
- ○ 250 g (9 oz) live yoghurt
- ○ 150 g (5½ oz) Greek yoghurt
- ○ 445 ml (15 fl oz) kefir milk
- ○ 5 eggs + 1 egg white

Vegetables

- ○ 150 g (5½ oz) spinach
- ○ 1 small cauliflower
- ○ 1 sweet potato + 1 ordinary potato
- ○ 150 g (5½ oz) purple potatoes
- ○ 2 purple eggplants (aubergines)
- ○ 100 g (3½ oz) chestnut or button mushrooms
- ○ 2 red bell peppers (capsicums)
- ○ 2 green zucchini (courgettes) + 70 g (2½ oz) zucchini
- ○ 2 yellow zucchini (courgettes)
- ○ 100 g (3½ oz) mixed salad leaves (rocket/arugula, spinach)
- ○ handful of rocket (arugula)
- ○ handful of salad cress
- ○ baby salad leaves
- ○ 150 g (5½ oz) cavolo nero
- ○ 150 g (5½ oz) cabbage
- ○ 150 g (5½ oz) silverbeet (Swiss chard)
- ○ 6 asparagus spears
- ○ 1 avocado
- ○ 1 tomato
- ○ 6 garlic cloves
- ○ 2 spring (green) onions
- ○ 1 small red onion
- ○ 3 tbsp soffritto (red onion, carrot, celery)
- ○ 1 small carrot
- ○ 1 bouquet garni of parsley, thyme, sage
- ○ 4 tbsp parsley
- ○ 15 g (½ oz) basil leaves
- ○ 1 tbsp dill
- ○ 1 small bunch of thyme

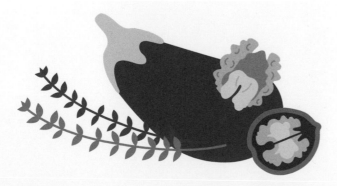

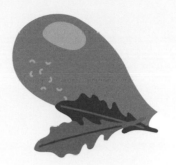

In the Storecupboard

- ○ 3 rye bread slices
- ○ 1 sourdough bread slice + 150 g (5½ oz) stale sourdough
- ○ 2 wholemeal tortillas
- ○ 100 g (3½ oz) green or brown lentils
- ○ 90 g (3 oz) spelt + spelt or barley to serve
- ○ 100 g (3½ oz) quinoa
- ○ 150 g (5½ oz) wholemeal couscous
- ○ 50 g (½ cup) rolled (porridge) oats + 1 tsp blitzed oats
- ○ 280 g (10 oz) granola
- ○ 200 g (7 oz) canned cannellini beans
- ○ 30 g (1 oz) Kalamata olives
- ○ 30 g (1 oz) walnuts
- ○ 4 g (¼ oz) pine nuts
- ○ 1 tbsp mixed nuts
- ○ 2 tsp mixed seeds
- ○ 4 tbsp chia seeds
- ○ wholemeal buckwheat flour
- ○ oat flour
- ○ extra virgin olive oil
- ○ rapeseed oil
- ○ maple syrup
- ○ honey
- ○ caster (superfine) sugar
- ○ red wine & white wine vinegar
- ○ balsamic vinegar
- ○ sumac
- ○ paprika
- ○ mixed spice
- ○ acai powder
- ○ baking powder

Fridge & Freezer Products

- ○ 50 g (1¾ oz) frozen edamame beans
- ○ 100 g (3½ oz) frozen mixed berries
- ○ 150 g (5½ oz) salmon fillet
- ○ 70 g (2½ oz) smoked salmon
- ○ 150 g (5½ oz) flank steak
- ○ 4 skin-on chicken thighs
- ○ 50 g (1¾ oz) tempeh
- ○ 600 ml (20½ fl oz) vegetable stock
- ○ 2 tbsp pickled cucumber
- ○ 75 g (2¾ oz) kimchi
- ○ 1 tbsp miso paste
- ○ 50 g (1¾ oz) silken tofu

Monday

The chia jam is not only great on toast, but it can be swirled through porridge or in yoghurt. This recipe works well with any juicy fruits like berries or peaches, apricots and cherries.

Breakfast

CHIA JAM ON RYE TOAST

SERVES: 1
PREPARATION: 5 MINUTES
COOK: 5 MINUTES

500 g (1 lb 2 oz) fresh raspberries
1 tablespoon lemon juice
4 tablespoons honey
4 tablespoons chia seeds
1 large slice rye bread

Cook fruit in a small saucepan over medium heat for 5 minutes, or until it breaks down. Remove from heat, mash fruit with back of a spatula, then add lemon juice and honey. Stir in chia seeds and mix to combine. Leave to set for about 5 minutes. Toast rye bread and spread with a dollop of chia jam.

Lunch

MOZZARELLA & ZUCCHINI SALAD WITH PESTO

SERVES: 1
PREPARATION: 5 MINUTES
COOK: 0 MINUTES

½ garlic clove
pinch of salt
15 g (½ oz) basil leaves
4 g (¼ oz) pine nuts
15 g (½ oz) parmesan, grated
25 ml (¾ fl oz) extra virgin olive oil
1 each green and yellow zucchini (courgettes), thinly sliced
1 small mozzarella ball, torn

For pesto, put garlic and salt into a mortar and start crushing until creamy consistency. Add basil and crush leaves by rotating pestle until a green liquid comes out. Add pine nuts and parmesan and reduce to a cream. To make pesto creamier, while stirring with pestle, add oil in a steady stream until combined. Put zucchini and mozzarella onto a plate, drizzle over pesto sauce and toss to combine. Serve.

Dinner

BAKED SWEET POTATO WITH WHIPPED FETA & SUMAC

SERVES: 1
PREPARATION: 5 MINUTES
COOK: 1 HOUR

1 sweet potato
50 g (1¾ oz) feta, crumbled
40 g (1½ oz) live yoghurt (page 66)
½ teaspoon sumac
1 teaspoon extra virgin olive oil
salt and pepper
1 tablespoon kimchi (page 64)

Preheat oven to 220°C (430°F). Prick sweet potato all over with a fork and bake for 1 hour, or until golden on outside and soft inside. In a small bowl, cream together feta and yoghurt and season with salt and pepper. Top potato with whipped feta, sprinkle with sumac, drizzle over oil and add kimchi. Serve.

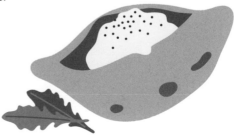

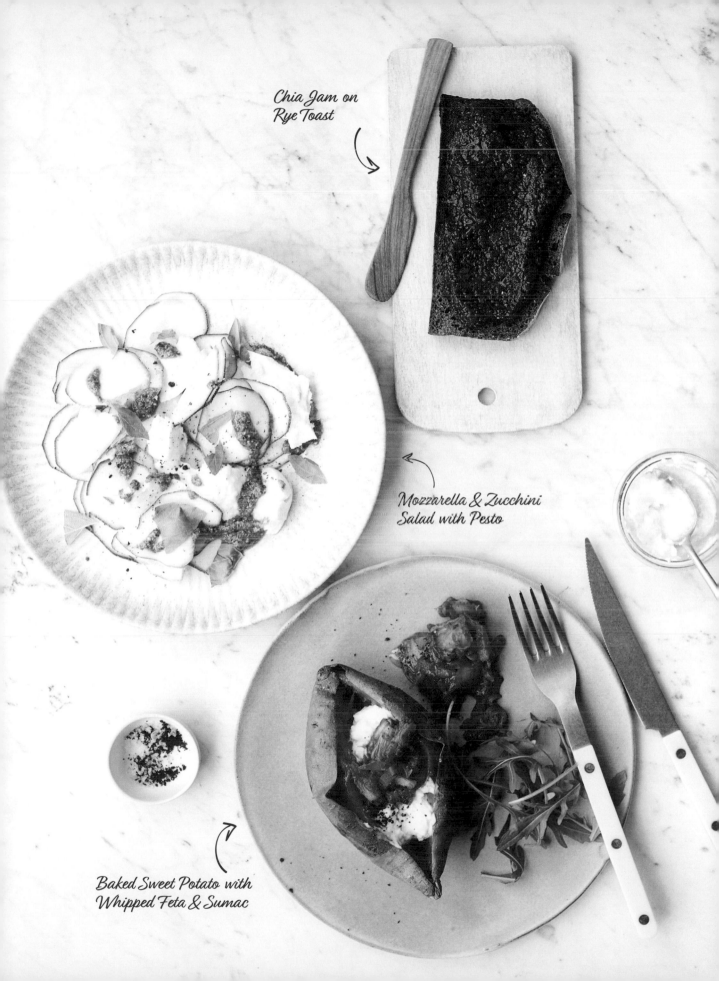

Chia Jam on Rye Toast

Mozzarella & Zucchini Salad with Pesto

Baked Sweet Potato with Whipped Feta & Sumac

Tuesday

A traditional Breton dish, this savoury pancake is a perfect healthy lunch burst with antioxidants and fibre from the buckwheat and vitamins and protein from the spinach.

Breakfast

LIVE YOGHURT PARFAIT

SERVES: 1
PREPARATION: 5 MINUTES
COOK: 0 MINUTES

150 g (5½ oz) live yoghurt (page 66)
1 teaspoon honey
2 tablespoons chia jam (page 112)
2 tablespoons granola (page 72)

Mix yoghurt and honey together in a bowl. In a small jar, alternate layers of yoghurt and jam, finishing with granola.

Lunch

SPINACH & GOAT'S CHEESE BUCKWHEAT GALETTE

SERVES: 1
PREPARATION: 5 MINUTES
COOK: 15 MINUTES

2 tablespoons extra virgin olive oil
1 garlic clove, chopped
50 g (1¾ oz) spinach, chopped
30 g (1 oz) goat's cheese, crumbled
80 g (2¾ oz) wholemeal buckwheat flour
1 egg, whisked
300 ml (10 fl oz) kefir milk
40 g (1½ oz) butter
salt and pepper

Heat 1 tablespoon oil in a frying pan over medium heat and fry garlic for 2 minutes. Add spinach and stir for 3 minutes. Remove from heat, season and fold in cheese. Set aside. Beat flour, egg, half the kefir and a pinch of salt together in a bowl to a smooth paste, then add remaining kefir to loosen mixture. Melt butter and stir into batter. Lightly oil a frying pan with 1 teaspoon oil and heat over medium–high heat. Spoon in half of the batter and cook for 3 minutes. Spread over some of filling, leaving a 2 cm (¾ in) border, then fold over edges leaving centre exposed and cook for 2 minutes. Remove and repeat with remaining batter. Serve.

Dinner

GRILLED EGGPLANT & LENTIL SALAD

SERVES: 1
PREPARATION: 5 MINUTES
COOK: 30 MINUTES

1 purple eggplant (aubergine), thickly sliced
2 tablespoons extra virgin olive oil
1 garlic clove, very finely chopped
1 tablespoon soffritto (finely chopped red onion, carrot, celery)
100 g (3½ oz) green or brown lentils
50 g (1¾ oz) mixed salad (rocket/ arugula, spinach)
salt and pepper

Preheat oven to 180°C (350°F). Place eggplant on a baking tray, drizzle with ½ tablespoon oil, garlic and a pinch of salt and bake for 25 minutes. Heat 1 tablespoon oil in a saucepan over medium heat and cook soffritto for 3 minutes. Add lentils, cover with water and cook for 25 minutes, or until all water has evaporated. Transfer lentils to a plate, add salad, remaining ½ tablespoon oil, season to taste and mix. Scatter over eggplant and mix slightly. Serve.

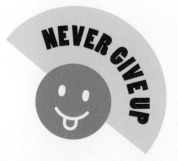
NEVER GIVE UP

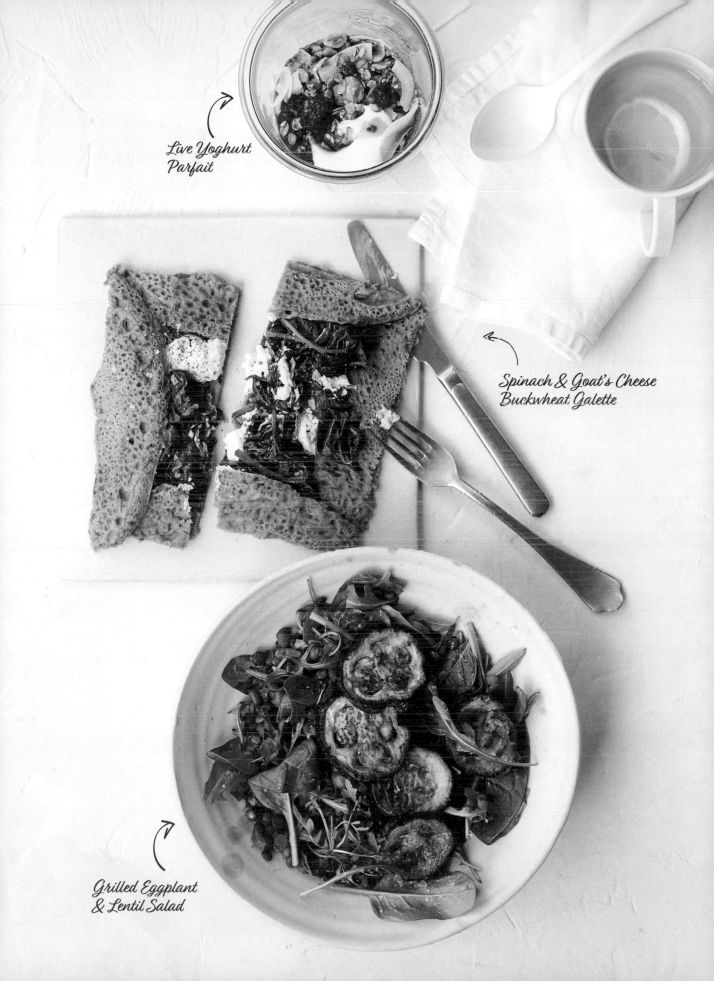

Live Yoghurt Parfait

Spinach & Goat's Cheese Buckwheat Galette

Grilled Eggplant & Lentil Salad

Wednesday

This classic Italian soup for lunch elevates beans and vegetables to another level, Ribollita, in Italian 'twice-boiled', means that the next day the soup is even tastier.

Breakfast

ACAI BOWL

SERVES: 1
PREPARATION: 5 MINUTES
COOK: 0 MINUTES

80 ml (⅓ cup) kefir milk
150 g (5½ oz) Greek yoghurt
100 g (3½ oz) frozen mixed berries
1 banana, sliced
1½ tablespoons acai powder
1 tablespoon mixed nuts, toasted
1 tablespoon mixed fresh berries
1 teaspoon mixed seeds

In a blender, put kefir, yoghurt, berries, banana and acai powder and blend until smooth and creamy. Transfer to a bowl and top with nuts, fresh berries and seeds.

Lunch

RIBOLLITA

SERVES: 4
PREPARATION: 5 MINUTES
COOK: 45 MINUTES

2 tablespoons extra virgin olive oil
2 tablespoons soffritto (finely chopped carrot, celery, red onion)
1 potato, diced
150 g (5½ oz) cavolo nero, tough stems removed and leaves chopped
150 g (5½ oz) cabbage, tough stems removed and leaves chopped
150 g (5½ oz) silverbeet (Swiss chard), chopped
200 g (7 oz) canned cannellini beans, drained and rinsed
150 g (5½ oz) stale sourdough bread, roughly chopped
salt and pepper

Heat oil in a pan over medium heat and fry soffritto for 3 minutes. Add potato, cook for 2 minutes, then add cavolo nero, cabbage, silverbeet and 1 litre (4 cups) boiling water. In a blender, blend half of cannellini beans with 250 ml (1 cup) hot water, then pour into pan. Bring to the boil and cook for 30 minutes, stirring occasionally. Add remaining beans and bread, season with salt and pepper and cook for another 10 minutes until bread has softened and absorbed some of the liquid. Freeze or store in fridge for another day.

Dinner

SALMON FISHCAKES & PICKLE

SERVES: 1
PREPARATION: 35 MINUTES
COOK: 15 MINUTES

1 bouquet garni of parsley, thyme, sage
½ lemon, sliced
1 garlic clove, sliced
150 g (5½ oz) salmon fillet
150 g (5½ oz) purple potatoes, peeled and cut into 2 cm (¾ in) cubes
1 tablespoon oat flour
2 tablespoons extra virgin olive oil
salt and pepper
2 tablespoons pickled cucumber (page 74), baby salad leaves and lemon wedge, to serve

Combine bouquet garni, sliced lemon, garlic, a pinch of salt and 150 ml (5 fl oz) water in a large saucepan and bring to the boil. Add salmon and cook for 5 minutes. Remove from liquid, cool slightly, then flake salmon into a bowl. Cook potatoes in another pan of salted boiling water, drain, then mash with a fork. Add to salmon, together with flour and some of the herbs of the bouquet garni. Season and divide mixture into 3 fishcakes. Cover and rest in fridge for 30 minutes. Heat oil in a large frying pan and cook fishcakes for 3 minutes on each side. Serve with pickled cucumber, salad and lemon wedge.

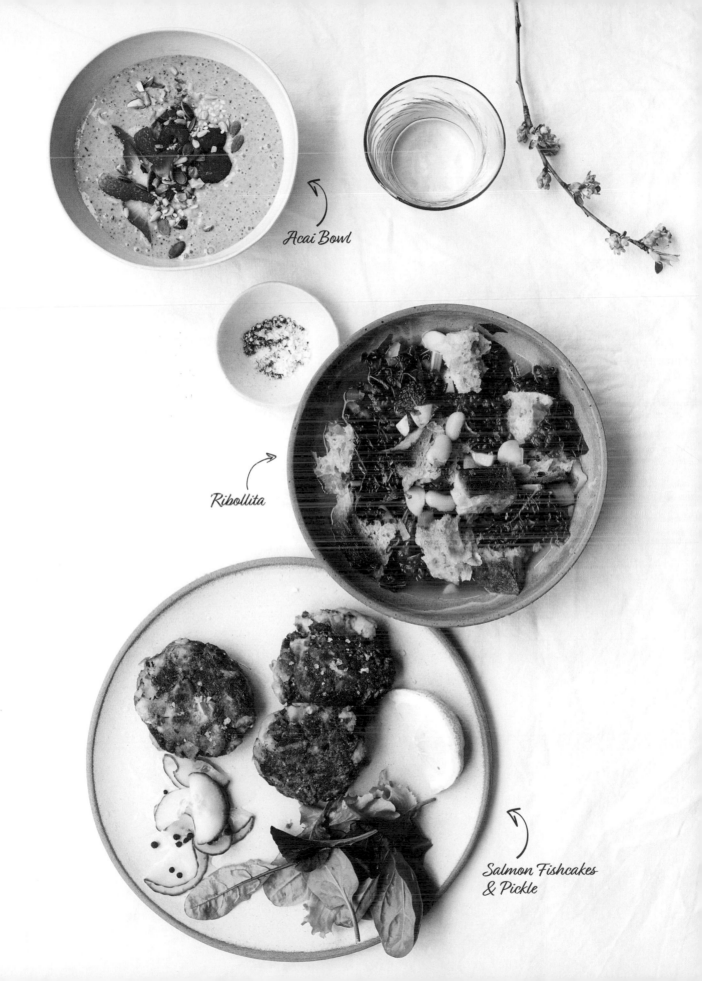

Acai Bowl

Ribollita

*Salmon Fishcakes
& Pickle*

Thursday

This dinner is economical, healthy and scrumptious.
Plus it is really quick to make if you have left-over cooked
barley, brown rice or quinoa from the night before.

Breakfast

BLUEBERRY GRANOLA COOKIES

MAKES: 12
PREPARATION: 5 MINUTES
COOK: 20 MINUTES

250 g (9 oz) granola (page 72)
50 g (1¾ oz) fresh or dried
    blueberries
1 egg white
1 tablespoon caster (superfine) sugar

Preheat oven to 170°C (340°F).
Combine granola and blueberries
in a bowl. In another bowl, beat egg
white with an electric mixer until
foamy. Add sugar and beat until soft
peaks form. Fold in granola mixture
until evenly coated. Using damp
hands, divide mixture into 12 balls,
then flatten each with palms of
hands. Put them onto a lined baking
tray and bake for about 20 minutes,
rotating baking tray halfway
through, until golden brown. Store
in an airtight container for up to
5 days.

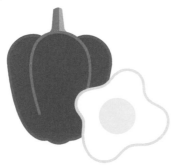

Lunch

ASPARAGUS & POACHED EGG

SERVES: 1
PREPARATION: 5 MINUTES
COOK: 10 MINUTES

1 large slice sourdough bread
6 asparagus spears
1 teaspoon extra virgin olive oil
1 teaspoon white wine vinegar
1 egg
salt and pepper

Heat a griddle pan over high heat,
toast bread and set aside. Chargrill
asparagus for 2 minutes on each
side, drizzle with oil, season with
salt and pepper and arrange on
bread. Bring a saucepan of salted
water to the boil, add vinegar and
reduce heat to simmer. Crack egg
into a small bowl, create a whirlpool
in simmering water with a spoon
and pour egg into centre. Cook for
2–3 minutes, then remove with a
slotted spoon and put on top of
asparagus. Sprinkle with pepper
and serve.

Dinner

STUFFED PEPPERS WITH SPELT & GOAT'S CHEESE

SERVES: 1
PREPARATION: 5 MINUTES
COOK: 25 MINUTES

2 tablespoons extra virgin olive oil
100 g (3½ oz) chestnut or button
    mushrooms, sliced
90 g (3 oz) cooked spelt
50 g (1¾ oz) goat's cheese, crumbled
1 teaspoon chopped parsley
1 red bell pepper (capsicum), halved
    lengthways and seeded
1 teaspoon blitzed rolled oat crumbs
salt and pepper
rocket (arugula), to serve

Preheat oven to 180°C (350°F). Heat
1 tablespoon oil in a large frying pan
and cook mushrooms for 5 minutes.
Season with salt and pepper and
place together with spelt in a bowl.
Add cheese and parsley and stir
to combine. Arrange bell pepper
halves, cut-side up, on a baking
tray and season with a pinch of salt.
Divide mixture evenly between
peppers, sprinkle with oat crumbs
and bake for 20 minutes until bell
peppers are soft and oats are golden.
Serve with rocket.

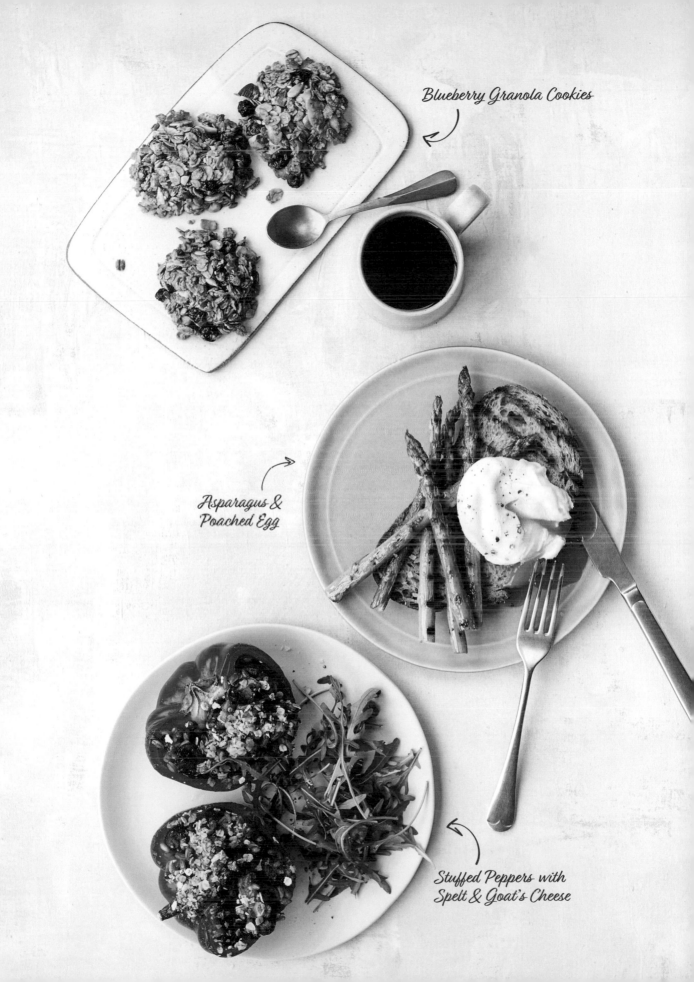

Blueberry Granola Cookies

*Asparagus &
Poached Egg*

*Stuffed Peppers with
Spelt & Goat's Cheese*

Friday

Easy to make, in less than 10 minutes, this lunch is filled with plant-based proteins and fibre. You can cook the quinoa ahead of time and freeze until ready to use.

Breakfast

SUPER GREEN FRITTERS

SERVES: 1 / MAKES: 4
PREPARATION: 15 MINUTES
COOK: 6 MINUTES

70 g (2½ oz) zucchini (courgettes), grated
60 g (2 oz) spinach, chopped
2 small eggs
1 tablespoon roughly chopped dill
1 tablespoon parmesan, grated
2 tablespoons oat flour
2 tablespoons rapeseed oil
50 g (1¾ oz) labneh
½ garlic clove, very finely chopped
salt and pepper
lemon wedge, to serve

Combine zucchini, spinach, eggs, dill and parmesan in a bowl. Season with salt and pepper, add flour and mix again. Rest for 10 minutes. Heat oil in a non-stick frying pan over medium heat. Using a large serving spoon, divide mixture into four equal portions and cook for 3 minutes on each side. Make dip by mixing labneh and garlic together in a bowl. Season to taste. Serve fritters with dip and lemon wedge.

Lunch

QUINOA SALAD WITH TEMPEH & CANDIED WALNUTS

SERVES: 1
PREPARATION: 5 MINUTES
COOK: 7 MINUTES

1 teaspoon butter
1 tablespoon caster (superfine) sugar
30 g (1 oz) walnuts
1 teaspoon balsamic vinegar
1½ tablespoons extra virgin olive oil
1 teaspoon honey
100 g (3½ oz) cooked quinoa
50 g (1¾ oz) tempeh, diced
50 g (1¾ oz) salad leaves of choice
salt

Melt butter and sugar in a frying pan, add walnuts and stir until completely coated. Arrange on a lined baking tray, separating them with a fork, then sprinkle with a pinch of salt and set aside. For dressing, mix vinegar, ½ tablespoon oil, honey and a pinch of salt together in a small bowl. Set aside. Heat remaining 1 tablespoon oil in a frying pan and cook tempeh, stirring, for 5 minutes, or until lightly browned. Mix all ingredients together in a bowl, drizzle with dressing and toss to combine.

Dinner

BEEF TACOS WITH KIMCHI SAUCE

SERVES: 1
PREPARATION: 35 MINUTES
COOK: 6 MINUTES

1 teaspoon balsamic vinegar
1 small red onion, very finely chopped
1 tablespoon extra virgin olive oil
½ teaspoon paprika
2 teaspoons chopped parsley
150 g (5½ oz) flank steak
1 tomato, diced
30 g (1 oz) kimchi, chopped (page 64)
2 wholemeal tortillas
small handful of spinach leaves

Combine vinegar, ½ onion, oil, paprika and 1 teaspoon parsley in a large, wide bowl, add steak, coat evenly, cover and rest in fridge for 30 minutes. For kimchi sauce, combine tomato, remaining onion, kimchi and remaining parsley in another bowl. Set aside. Preheat a griddle pan over medium heat and cook steak for 3 minutes on each side. Remove from pan, cover and rest for 5 minutes. Warm tortillas, cut steak into strips, put into tortilla and top with kimchi sauce and spinach. Serve.

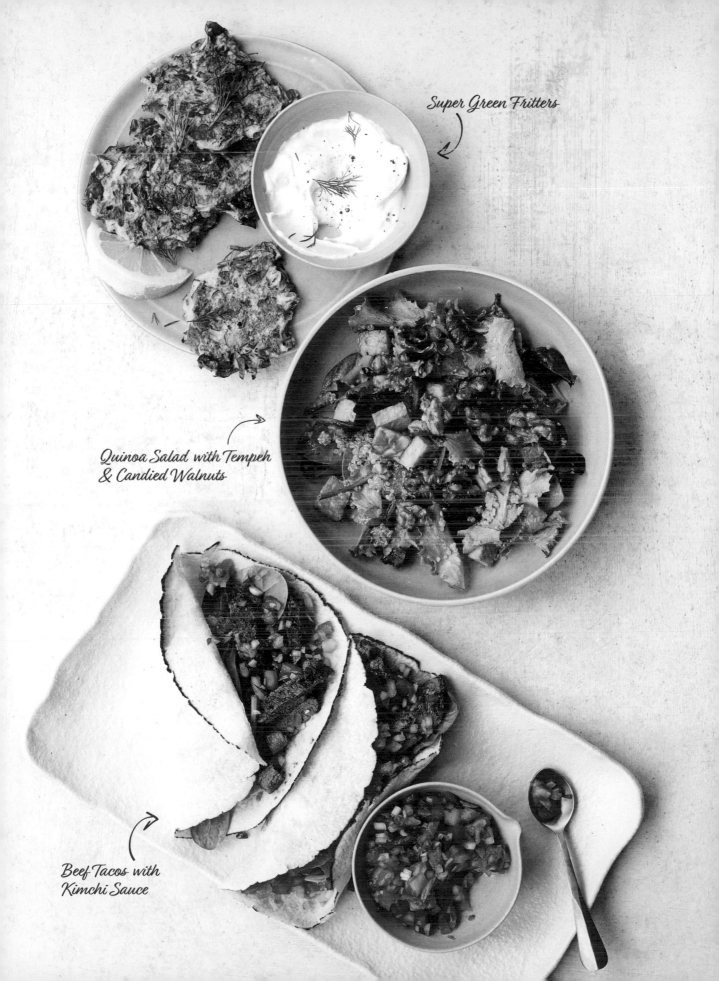

Super Green Fritters

Quinoa Salad with Tempeh & Candied Walnuts

Beef Tacos with Kimchi Sauce

Saturday

This creamy cauliflower soup for dinner can be made ahead of time and stored in the freezer. You can swap the cauliflower for the green and purple varieties, as well as the sweeter Romanesco cauliflower.

Breakfast

OAT BANANA PANCAKES WITH RASPBERRIES

SERVES: 1 / MAKES: 4
PREPARATION: 5 MINUTES
COOK: 5 MINUTES

65 ml (2¼ fl oz) kefir milk
1 egg, separated
1 small banana, roughly chopped
1 teaspoon baking powder
2 tablespoons maple syrup, plus extra to serve
50 g (½ cup) rolled (porridge) oats
1 teaspoon rapeseed oil
2 tablespoons raspberries

Mix kefir, egg yolk, banana, baking powder, 1 tablespoon maple syrup and oats in a blender. In a bowl, whisk egg white until frothy, then gently fold in oat mixture. Heat oil in a non-stick frying pan over medium heat, add 2 tablespoons of batter and cook for 1–2 minutes on each side. Repeat with remaining batter. Serve with syrup and raspberries.

Lunch

GRIDDLED VEGETABLES & FETA COUSCOUS

SERVES: 2
PREPARATION: 5 MINUTES
COOK: 20 MINUTES

1 each small green and yellow zucchini (courgette), sliced
1 small purple eggplant (aubergine), sliced
1 red bell pepper (capsicum), sliced
150 g (5½ oz) wholemeal couscous
2 tablespoons chopped parsley
2 tablespoons extra virgin olive oil
50 g (1¾ oz) feta, crumbled
1 tablespoon pomegranate seeds
salt and pepper

Heat a griddle pan over high heat and chargrill vegetables for 5–8 minutes until tender. Put couscous into a large bowl with 150 ml (5 fl oz) boiling water, cover and leave for 10–12 minutes until water is absorbed. Using a fork, fluff up couscous, add vegetables, parsley and oil. Season to taste and mix well. Spoon onto a plate and add feta and pomegranate seeds. Serve. Store leftovers in fridge for another time.

Dinner

CAULIFLOWER SOUP

SERVES: 1
PREPARATION: 5 MINUTES
COOK: 14 MINUTES

1 tablespoon extra virgin olive oil
1 garlic clove, sliced
1 teaspoon mixed spice
1 small cauliflower, cut into florets
300 ml (10 fl oz) vegetable stock
1 teaspoon chopped parsley
1 teaspoon toasted seeds
salt and pepper

Heat oil in a large saucepan over medium heat and cook garlic and spice for 1 minute. Add cauliflower and stir for 1 minute before adding stock. Bring to the boil, then simmer for 10 minutes, or until cauliflower is tender. Transfer to blender and blitz until creamy and smooth. Pour soup back into pan, season with salt and pepper and simmer for 2 minutes. Ladle into a bowl and sprinkle with parsley and seeds.

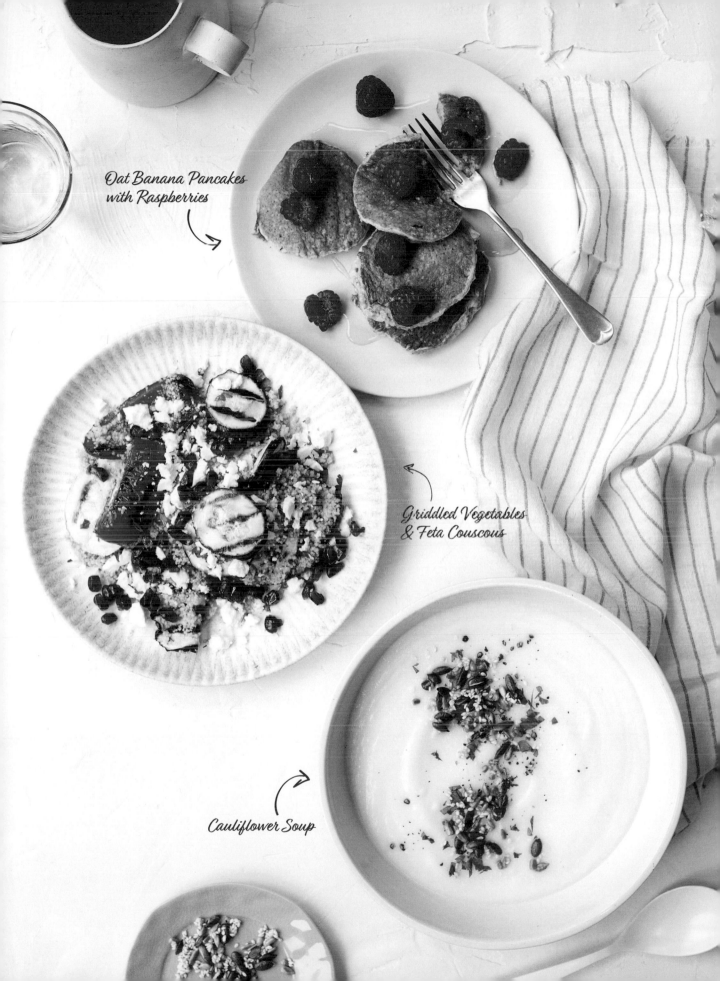

Oat Banana Pancakes
with Raspberries

Griddled Vegetables
& Feta Couscous

Cauliflower Soup

Sunday

A favourite option for many, this breakfast has the additional benefit of plant-based protein, fibre and other essential nutrients from the edamame beans.

Breakfast

AVOCADO & EDAMAME TOAST WITH SMOKED SALMON

SERVES: 1
PREPARATION: 5 MINUTES
COOK: 5 MINUTES

50 g (1¾ oz) frozen edamame beans, thawed
1 avocado
2 tablespoons live yoghurt (page 66)
1 tablespoon lemon juice
2 slices rye bread, toasted
70 g (2½ oz) smoked salmon
handful of salad cress
salt and pepper
lemon wedge, to serve

Steam edamame beans for 5 minutes, then blitz half in a blender with 2 tablespoons water. Scoop avocado flesh into a bowl, add blended edamame, yoghurt and lemon juice and mix with a fork. Fold in remaining edamame, season with salt and pepper and divide between toasted bread. Add smoked salmon, sprinkle over some pepper and top with cress. Serve with lemon wedge.

Lunch

ONE-POT MISO SOUP

SERVES: 1
PREPARATION: 5 MINUTES
COOK: 12 MINUTES

300 ml (10 fl oz) vegetable stock
1 garlic clove, sliced
2 spring (green) onions, sliced
1 small carrot, julienned
50 g (1¾ oz) silken tofu, diced
1 tablespoon miso paste

Bring stock to the boil in a large saucepan. Add garlic, spring onions and carrot, cover with a lid and simmer for 5 minutes. Add tofu and simmer for 3 minutes, then turn off heat. In a small bowl, loosen up miso paste with 1 tablespoon stock, then pour it into pan. Serve.

Dinner

PAN-ROASTED CHICKEN WITH OLIVES, LEMON & THYME

SERVES: 2
PREPARATION: 35 MINUTES
COOK: 30 MINUTES

4 chicken thighs, skin-on
3 tablespoons red wine vinegar
2 tablespoons extra virgin olive oil
30 g (1 oz) Kalamata olives, pitted
1 small lemon, sliced
1 small bunch of thyme
salt and pepper
1 portion cooked spelt or pearl barley, to serve

Put chicken into a shallow dish, add vinegar and oil, cover and marinate in fridge for 30 minutes. Heat a frying pan over high heat and sear chicken thighs, skin-side down, for 5 minutes. Turn over and cook for about 10 minutes. Add olives, lemon and thyme, cook for 10–15 minutes until chicken is cooked. Season and serve with spelt. Store leftovers in fridge for later.

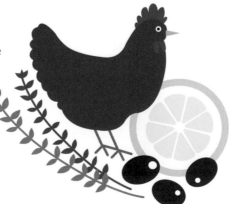

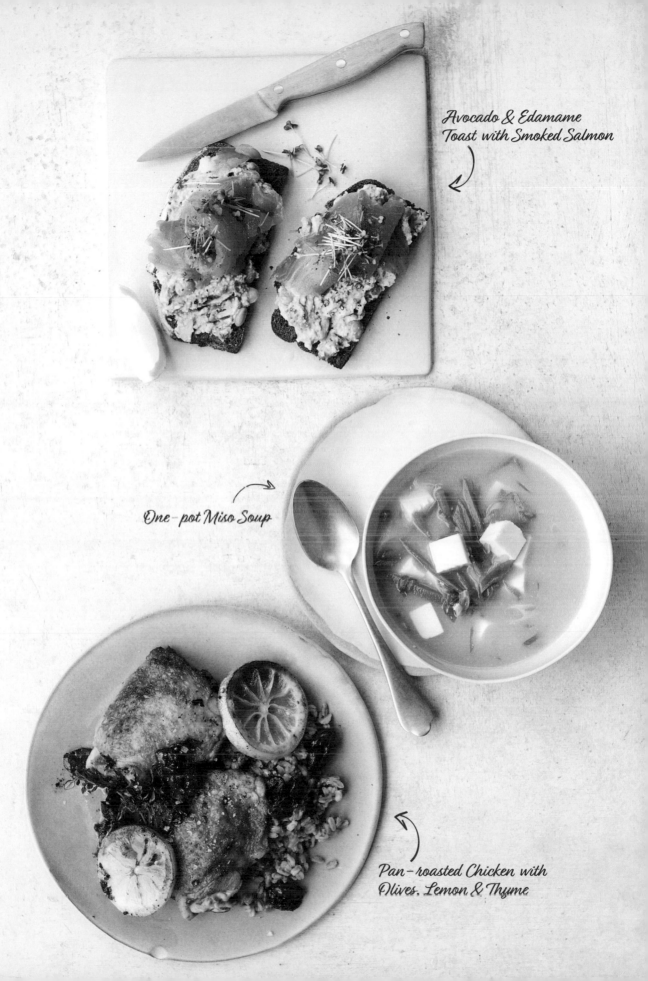

Avocado & Edamame Toast with Smoked Salmon

One-pot Miso Soup

Pan-roasted Chicken with Olives, Lemon & Thyme

Fruit

- ○ 4½ bananas
- ○ 35 g (1¼ oz) mixed berries
- ○ 2 Medjool dates
- ○ 1 pear
- ○ ½ apple
- ○ 50 g (⅓ cup) blueberries
- ○ 25 g (1 oz) pomegranate seeds
- ○ ½ lime
- ○ 2 lemons + lemon wedge

Vegetables

- ○ 5 cherry tomatoes
- ○ 250 g (9 oz) ripe tomatoes + extra to garnish
- ○ 150 g (5½ oz) small beetroot (beets)
- ○ 2 red bell peppers (capsicums)
- ○ 1 small cucumber
- ○ handful of rocket (arugula)
- ○ 100 g (3½ oz) mixed salad leaves
- ○ 100 g (3½ oz) Jerusalem artichokes
- ○ ½ small radicchio
- ○ 400 g (14 oz) sweet potatoes
- ○ 200 g (7 oz) rainbow chard
- ○ 3 kale leaves
- ○ 4 small red onions
- ○ 3 garlic cloves
- ○ 1 spring (green) onion
- ○ 2 tbsp parsley
- ○ 1 bouquet garni with thyme, rosemary, sage, bay leaves
- ○ 1 tbsp mint
- ○ 1 tsp chives
- ○ 3 thyme sprigs
- ○ 1½ tbsp coriander (cilantro)

Eggs & Dairy Products

- ○ 510 ml (17 fl oz) kefir milk
- ○ 250 ml (1 cup) milk of your choice
- ○ 55 g (2 oz) live yoghurt
- ○ 165 g (6 oz) Greek yoghurt
- ○ 15 g (½ oz) parmesan
- ○ 1½ tbsp butter
- ○ 50 g (1¾ oz) feta
- ○ 100 g (3½ oz) halloumi cheese
- ○ 25 g (1 oz) Taleggio cheese
- ○ 6 eggs

In the Storecupboard

- [ ] 1 large slice rye bread
- [ ] 2 slices sourdough bread
- [ ] 80 g (2¾ oz) sourdough bread for crostini
- [ ] 70 g (2½ oz) buckwheat noodles
- [ ] 180 g (6½ oz) rolled (porridge) oats
- [ ] 100 g (3½ oz) canned borlotti (cranberry) beans
- [ ] 250 g (9 oz) mixed dried beans
- [ ] 150 g (5½ oz) canned chickpeas (garbanzo beans)
- [ ] 100 g (3½ oz) canned brown or green lentils
- [ ] 150 g (5½ oz) dried broad (fava) beans
- [ ] 100 ml (3½ fl oz) canned coconut milk
- [ ] 80 g (2¾ oz) quinoa
- [ ] 30 g (1 oz) bulgur wheat
- [ ] 80 g (2¾ oz) spelt
- [ ] 80 g (2¾ oz) freekeh
- [ ] 15 g (½ oz) whole almonds
- [ ] 1 tsp toasted mixed nuts
- [ ] 2½ tbsp chia seeds
- [ ] 1 tbsp hazelnuts
- [ ] 200 g (7 oz) mixed seeds
- [ ] ½ tbsp sesame seeds
- [ ] 50 g (1¾ oz) almond flour
- [ ] 50 g (⅓ cup) wholemeal (whole-wheat) flour
- [ ] 300 g (10½ oz) spelt flour
- [ ] 20 g (¾ oz) cornflour (cornstarch)
- [ ] extra virgin olive oil
- [ ] rapeseed oil
- [ ] 75 ml (2½ fl oz) coconut oil

- [ ] 15 g (½ oz) green olives
- [ ] 10 g (¼ oz) salted capers
- [ ] Dijon mustard
- [ ] 1 tbsp white wine
- [ ] apple cider vinegar
- [ ] red wine vinegar
- [ ] balsamic vinegar
- [ ] honey
- [ ] maple syrup
- [ ] caster (superfine) sugar
- [ ] mirin
- [ ] chilli sauce
- [ ] dark chocolate chips
- [ ] soy sauce
- [ ] baking powder
- [ ] chilli flakes
- [ ] ground turmeric
- [ ] ground cinnamon
- [ ] curry powder
- [ ] spirulina powder

Fridge & Freezer Products

- [ ] 200 g (7 oz) skinless boneless chicken breasts
- [ ] 150 g (5½ oz) tuna steak
- [ ] 1 salmon fillet
- [ ] 80 g (2¾ oz) firm tofu
- [ ] 80 g (2¾ oz) silken tofu
- [ ] 1.2 litres (41 fl oz) vegetable stock
- [ ] 2 tbsp pickles (gherkins)
- [ ] 150 g (5½ oz) frozen mixed berries

Monday

Beetroot is part of the same family as spinach and, being low in fat, full of antioxidants, vitamins and minerals, they can be called health-food giants.

Breakfast

SPICY SCRAMBLED EGGS ON RYE TOAST

SERVES: 1
PREPARATION: 5 MINUTES
COOK: 8 MINUTES

2 eggs
½ teaspoon ground turmeric
1 large slice rye bread
1 teaspoon butter
5 cherry tomatoes, halved
½ teaspoon chilli flakes
1 tablespoon chopped coriander (cilantro)

In a small bowl, mix eggs and turmeric together. Heat a small frying pan over low heat, toast bread and set aside. In same pan, add butter, tomatoes and chilli and cook for 3 minutes. Add eggs and cook, stirring, for 2–3 minutes. Serve eggs on toasted bread sprinkled with coriander leaves.

Lunch

SLOW-COOKED BEETROOT WITH FETA

SERVES: 1
PREPARATION: 5 MINUTES
COOK: 1 HOUR

150 g (5½ oz) small beetroot (beets), halved
1 small red onion, cut into wedges
¼ teaspoon chilli flakes
1 tablespoon red wine vinegar
1 tablespoon extra virgin olive oil
50 g (1¾ oz) feta, sliced
salt and pepper

Preheat oven to 180°C (350°F). Scrunch and wet 2 pieces of baking paper. Put beetroot, onion, chilli and vinegar into a roasting pan lined with 1 piece wet baking paper, drizzle with oil, season with salt and pepper and cover with other piece of paper. Bake for 1 hour, or until tender. Remove top paper and sprinkle over feta.

Dinner

SPICY FAJITA BUDDHA BOWL WITH BEANS

SERVES: 1
PREPARATION: 5 MINUTES
COOK: 10 MINUTES

1 tablespoon extra virgin olive oil
1 small red bell pepper (capsicum), sliced
1 small red onion, sliced
50 g (1¾ oz) canned borlotti (cranberry) beans, drained and rinsed
¼ teaspoon chilli flakes
50 g (¼ cup) quinoa, cooked
½ tablespoon chopped coriander (cilantro)
juice of ½ lime
50 g (1¾ oz) mixed salad leaves, chopped
salt and pepper

Heat oil in a medium saucepan over medium heat and cook red bell pepper and onion for 5 minutes. Season and add beans and chilli with 1 tablespoon water. Mix well and cook for another 5 minutes. Mix quinoa, coriander and lime juice together in a bowl. Put salad leaves in a serving bowl, then top with quinoa, red pepper and bean mixture and serve.

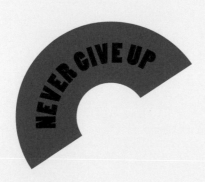
NEVER GIVE UP

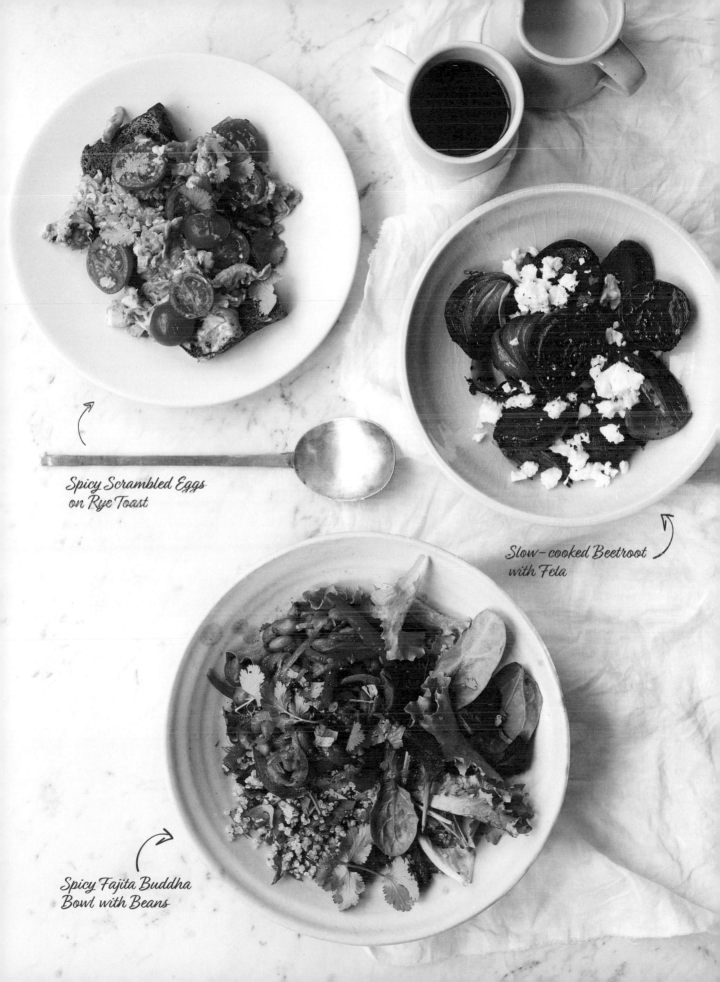

Spicy Scrambled Eggs
on Rye Toast

Slow-cooked Beetroot
with Feta

Spicy Fajita Buddha
Bowl with Beans

Tuesday

Onions are full of antioxidants and the pairing with the protein, fibre and mineral content of the sweet potatoes, makes this dinner unbeatable.

Breakfast

KEFIR, BANANA & BERRIES SMOOTHIE

SERVES: 1
PREPARATION: 5 MINUTES
COOK: 0 MINUTES

150 ml (5 fl oz) kefir milk
½ banana, sliced
35 g (1¼ oz) mixed berries
15 g (½ oz) whole almonds, toasted
2 Medjool dates, stoned
   and chopped

Put all ingredients into a blender and blitz until smooth. Serve.

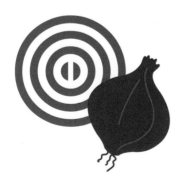

Lunch

JERUSALEM ARTICHOKE & POACHED CHICKEN SALAD

SERVES: 1
PREPARATION: 5 MINUTES
COOK: 30 MINUTES

100 g (3½ oz) Jerusalem artichokes,
   cut into chunks
4 tablespoons extra virgin olive oil
1 pear, cut in half lengthways,
   then into 6 wedges, stalks
   and core removed
1 skinless, boneless chicken
   breast fillet
1 thyme sprig
½ lemon, sliced
1 teaspoon balsamic vinegar
1 tablespoon honey
salt and pepper

Preheat oven to 200°C (400°F). Put artichokes into a roasting pan, toss with 1 tablespoon oil, season and roast for 25 minutes. Add pear and roast for another 5 minutes. Put chicken, thyme and lemon into a large saucepan, cover with cold water, bring to the boil, then simmer for 10 minutes, or until cooked. Drain well and when cool enough, shred chicken into pieces. Set aside. For dressing, whisk remaining 3 tablespoons oil, vinegar and honey together in a bowl. Season. Drizzle dressing over artichokes, toss and add chicken.

Dinner

SWEET POTATO & RED ONION SOUP

SERVES: 2
PREPARATION: 5 MINUTES
COOK: 20 MINUTES

1 tablespoon extra virgin olive oil
1 small red onion, sliced
400 g (14 oz) sweet potatoes, peeled
   and diced
400 ml (13½ fl oz) vegetable stock
1 teaspoon toasted mixed nuts
1 teaspoon chopped chives
1 tablespoon Greek yoghurt
salt and pepper
sourdough bread, to serve

Heat oil in a large saucepan over medium heat and cook onion for 3 minutes. Add sweet potatoes, cook for 2 minutes, then add stock and simmer for 15 minutes. Blend soup with a stick blender and season to taste. Ladle soup into a bowl, sprinkle over nuts, chives and add dollop of yoghurt. Serve with bread. Store leftovers in fridge for another time.

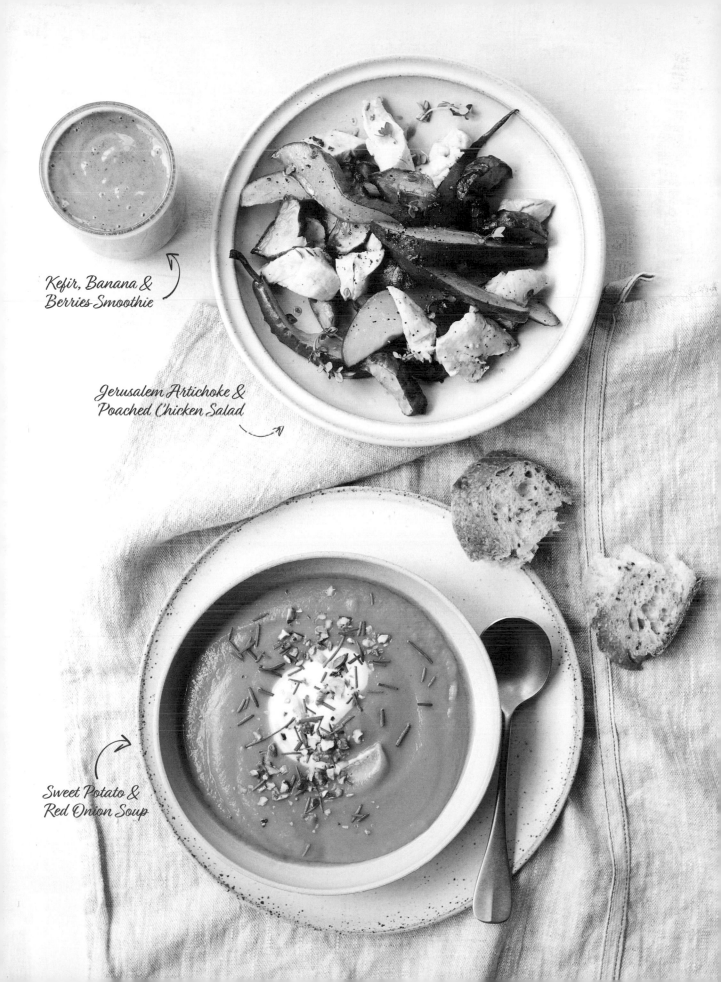

Kefir, Banana &
Berries Smoothie

Jerusalem Artichoke &
Poached Chicken Salad

Sweet Potato &
Red Onion Soup

Wednesday

Overnight oats can be stored in the fridge for up to five days, which makes this an ideal breakfast meal prep to make on Sunday night to enjoy during the week.

Breakfast

EASY OVERNIGHT OATS

SERVES: 1
PREPARATION: 5 MINUTES + OVERNIGHT
COOK: 0 MINUTES

50 g (½ cup) rolled (porridge) oats
1 teaspoon chia seeds
50 ml (1¾ fl oz) kefir milk
25 g (1 oz) live yoghurt (page 66)
1 teaspoon maple syrup
fruit, such as kiwi fruit and blueberries, to serve (optional)

Combine oats and chia seeds in a bowl. Add kefir, yoghurt and maple syrup, stir to combine, cover and rest overnight in fridge. In morning, stir and serve with maple syrup and fresh fruit, if desired.

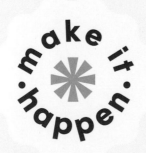

Lunch

GRILLED HALLOUMI & POMEGRANATE TABBOULEH

SERVES: 1
PREPARATION: 20 MINUTES
COOK: 5 MINUTES

30 g (1 oz) bulgur wheat
grated zest and juice of ½ lemon
1 tablespoon extra virgin olive oil
50 g (1¾ oz) canned chickpeas (garbanzo beans), drained and rinsed
1 tablespoon chopped parsley
1 tablespoon chopped mint
25 g (1 oz) pomegranate seeds
100 g (3½ oz) halloumi cheese, sliced
salt and pepper

Put the bulgur wheat into a heatproof bowl with 100 ml (3½ fl oz) boiling water, cover and leave for 15 minutes, or until tender. Drain and return to the bowl. Whisk lemon zest and juice with oil in another bowl and add to bulgur together with chickpeas, herbs and half the pomegranate seeds. Season with salt and pepper. Put a frying pan over medium heat and cook halloumi for 2 minutes on each side. Top tabbouleh with halloumi and sprinkle with remaining pomegranate seeds.

Dinner

LENTIL & CHICKPEA BURGERS WITH CUCUMBER PICKLE

SERVES: 1
PREPARATION: 35 MINUTES
COOK: 8 MINUTES

200 g (7 oz) canned mixed lentils and chickpeas (garbanzo beans), drained and rinsed
1 teaspoon ground turmeric
1 teaspoon chopped parsley
grated zest and juice of ½ lemon
1 egg
pinch of salt
20 g (¾ oz) cornflour (cornstarch)
1 tablespoon rapeseed oil
2 tablespoons pickles (gherkins), rocket (arugula) and lemon wedge, to serve

Blitz pulses, turmeric, parsley, lemon zest and juice, egg and salt together in a food processor until smooth. Transfer to a bowl, mix in cornstarch and form into 2 burgers. Chill for 30 minutes. Heat oil in a large frying pan over medium heat and fry burgers for 4 minutes on each side, or until cooked. Serve with pickles, rocket and lemon wedge.

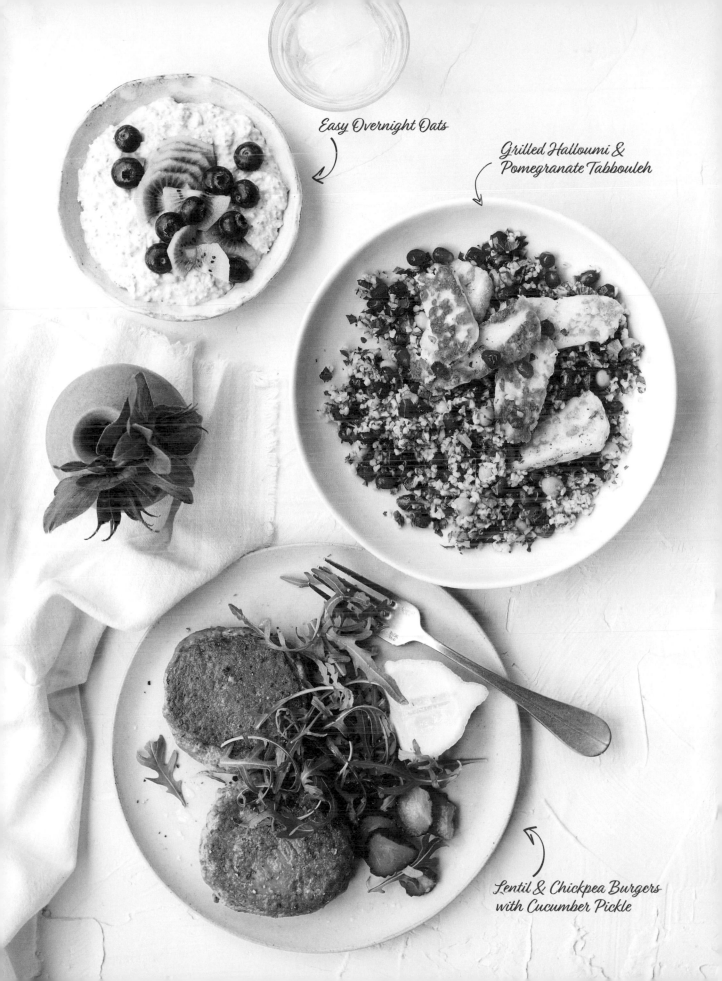

Easy Overnight Oats

*Grilled Halloumi &
Pomegranate Tabbouleh*

*Lentil & Chickpea Burgers
with Cucumber Pickle*

Thursday

Broad beans are loaded with nutrients and are delicious prepared with vegetables in stews and soups. You can store the rest of the dinner in the fridge for another time.

Breakfast

BLUEBERRY & SPIRULINA SHAKE

SERVES: 1
PREPARATION: 5 MINUTES
COOK: 0 MINUTES

80 g (2¾ oz) silken tofu, diced
50 g (⅓ cup) blueberries
250 ml (1 cup) kefir milk
1 teaspoon maple syrup
1 teaspoon spirulina powder

Put all the ingredients into a blender and blitz until smooth. Serve.

Lunch

SEARED TUNA WITH CAPERS & OLIVE SALSA

SERVES: 1
PREPARATION: 5 MINUTES
COOK: 6 MINUTES

15 g (½ oz) green olives, stoned and chopped
10 g (¼ oz) salted capers, rinsed, drained and chopped
2 tablespoons extra virgin olive oil
1 teaspoon chopped parsley
1 teaspoon lemon juice
¼ teaspoon chilli flakes
150 g (5½ oz) tuna steak
salt and pepper

Combine the olives, capers, 1 tablespoon oil, parsley, lemon juice and chilli in a large bowl and season to taste. Heat remaining oil in a non-stick frying pan and sear tuna steak for 3 minutes on each side. Serve tuna with olive sauce.

Dinner

BROAD BEAN STEW

SERVES: 2
PREPARATION: 5 MINUTES + OVERNIGHT
COOK: 45 MINUTES

150 g (5½ oz) dried broad (fava) beans
2 tablespoons extra virgin olive oil
1 garlic clove, chopped
½ teaspoon chilli flakes
200 g (7 oz) rainbow chard, chopped
salt and pepper
1 slice sourdough bread, toasted, to serve

Soak broad beans in a bowl of water overnight. Next day, drain well, rinse and put into a large saucepan. Cover with water and cook for 30 minutes. Heat 1 tablespoon oil in a frying pan over medium heat and fry garlic and chilli for 1 minute. Add to beans, then add chard and cook for 15 minutes, adding more water, if necessary. Season to taste, drizzle with remaining oil and serve with toasted bread.

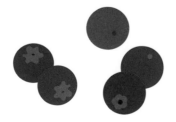

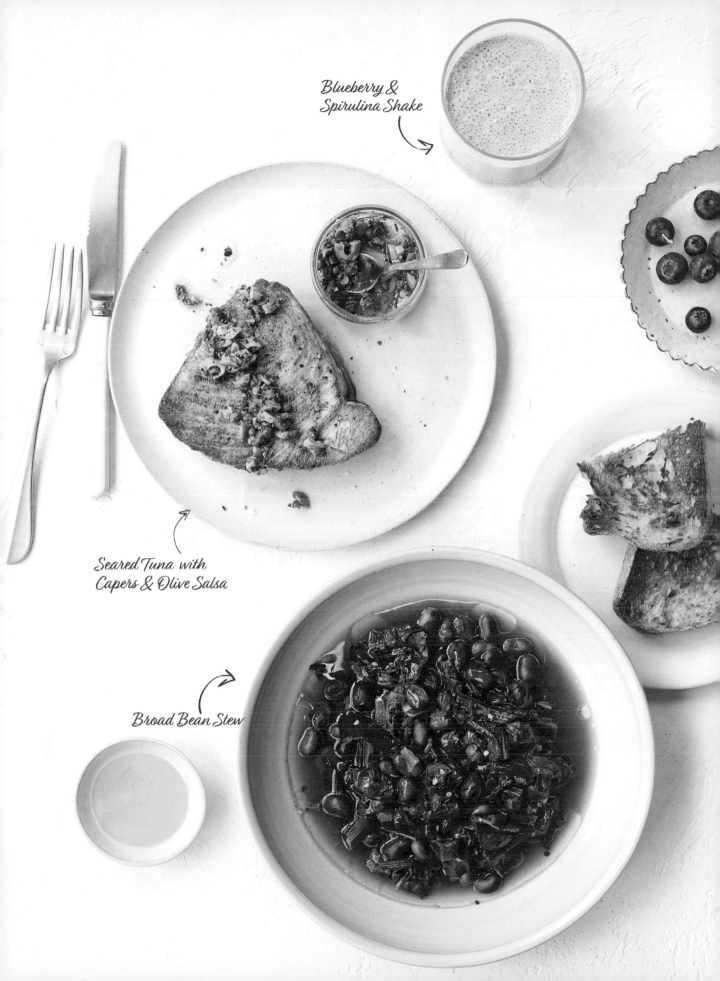

Blueberry &
Spirulina Shake

Seared Tuna with
Capers & Olive Salsa

Broad Bean Stew

Friday

This dinner is so simple to make and is the best way to use any left-over pulses you have in your storecupboard, Store the rest of the soup in the fridge for another time.

Breakfast

OVERNIGHT QUINOA, OAT, APPLE & HAZELNUTS

SERVES: 1
PREPARATION: 5 MINUTES
+ OVERNIGHT
COOK: 0 MINUTES

30 g (1 oz) quinoa, cooked
40 g (1½ oz) rolled (porridge) oats
1 teaspoon honey
½ teaspoon ground cinnamon
250 ml (1 cup) milk of your choice
½ apple, unpeeled, cored and
    chopped
1 tablespoon hazelnuts, chopped

To a wide-mouth mason jar, add quinoa, oats, honey and cinnamon. Top with milk, stir to combine, then cover with lid and chill in fridge overnight. In the morning, stir well before adding apple and hazelnuts.

Lunch

TOFU SKEWERS & FREEKEH SALAD

SERVES: 1
PREPARATION: 35 MINUTES
COOK: 5 MINUTES

1 tablespoon triple nut butter
    (page 70)
½ teaspoon curry powder
100 ml (3½ fl oz) coconut milk
80 g (2¾ oz) firm tofu, sliced into 4 cm
    (1½ in) cubes
½ red bell pepper (capsicum), sliced
    into 4 cm (1½ in) cubes
80 g (2¾ oz) freekeh, cooked
50 g (1¾ oz) mixed salad leaves

Mix butter, curry powder and coconut milk together thoroughly in a bowl. Stir in tofu and rest for 30 minutes. Remove tofu and thread onto metal skewers alternating with red pepper. In the bowl with left-over marinade, toss freekeh and salad leaves, then transfer to a plate. Heat a griddle pan over medium heat and cook tofu skewers for 2 minutes on each side. Serve on top of salad.

Dinner

MEDITERRANEAN SOUP

SERVES: 3
PREPARATION: 5 MINUTES
+ OVERNIGHT
COOK: 70 MINUTES

250 g (9 oz) mixed dried beans
    such as cannellini and borlotti
    (cranberry) beans, lentils and
    chickpeas (garbanzo beans)
1 tablespoon extra virgin olive oil,
    plus extra to drizzle
1 garlic clove, very finely chopped
500 ml (2 cups) vegetable stock
1 bouquet garni with thyme,
    rosemary, sage, bay leaves
salt and pepper
thyme sprigs, to garnish

Soak beans or pulses in a large bowl of cold water overnight. Next day, drain well and rinse. Heat oil in a large saucepan over medium heat and cook garlic for 1 minute. Add beans, stir, then cover with stock. Add bouquet garni, slowly bring to the boil, season to taste and simmer for about 1 hour, adding more stock, if necessary, until beans are soft. Once cooked, remove bouquet garni, drizzle with oil and garnish with thyme.

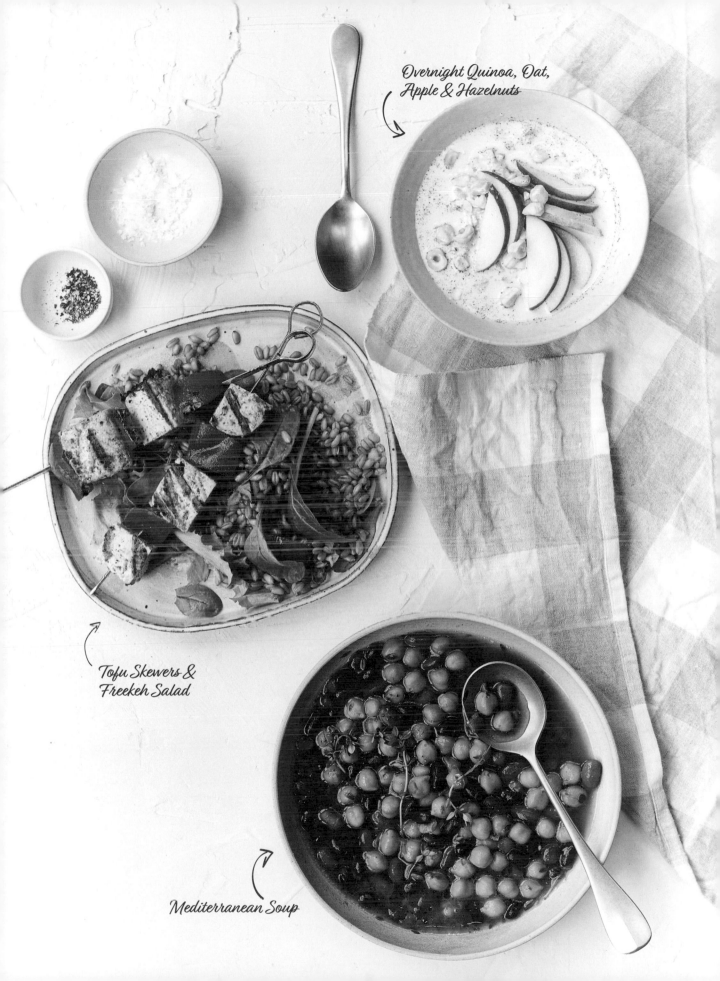

Overnight Quinoa, Oat,
Apple & Hazelnuts

Tofu Skewers &
Freekeh Salad

Mediterranean Soup

Saturday

Spelt is an ancient whole grain which contains a range of vitamins and minerals. It is also rich in fibre and is a hearty addition to the salad with its nutty, sweet flavour.

Breakfast

BREAKFAST BARS

SERVES: 1
PREPARATION: 5 MINUTES
COOK: 35 MINUTES

150 g (5½ oz) frozen mixed berries
100 ml (3½ fl oz) maple syrup
2 tablespoons chia seeds
1 egg
50 g (1¾ oz) almond flour
50 g (⅓ cup) wholemeal (whole-wheat) flour
90 g (3 oz) rolled (porridge) oats
75 ml (2½ fl oz) coconut oil, melted

Preheat oven to 180°C (350°F). Mix berries, 30 ml (1 fl oz) maple syrup, chia seeds and 1 tablespoon water in a saucepan and cook over medium heat for 5–8 minutes. Mix egg, flours, oats, coconut oil and remaining maple syrup together in a bowl. Set 30 g (1 oz) of mixture aside, then spread rest in a lined 15 cm (6 in) square baking tin. Cover with berry mix and sprinkle over reserved 30 g (1 oz) oat mixture. Bake for 25 minutes, or until golden brown. Cool before cutting into 6 bars. Store in an airtight container in fridge for 2–3 days.

Lunch

CHARRED CHICKEN & KALE CAESAR SALAD

SERVES: 1
PREPARATION: 5 MINUTES
COOK: 25 MINUTES

80 g (2¾ oz) sourdough bread, chopped
3 tablespoons extra virgin olive oil
¼ teaspoon sea salt
3 kale leaves, stems removed, leaves torn
100 g (3½ oz) skinless, boneless chicken breast
½ garlic clove, mashed
30 g (1 oz) live yoghurt (page 66)
1 teaspoon Dijon mustard
15 g (½ oz) shaved parmesan
salt and pepper

Preheat oven to 180°C (350°F). Toss bread with 1 tablespoon oil, sprinkle with salt, then spread out on a lined baking tray and bake for 10 minutes. Set aside. Put kale into a large bowl, drizzle with 1 tablespoon oil and season with salt and pepper. Arrange on a lined baking tray and bake for 15 minutes until crispy. Heat a frying pan over medium heat. Rub chicken with rest of oil, season and cook for 4 minutes on each side, or until fully cooked. Remove from pan, slice and set aside. For dressing, mix garlic, yoghurt and mustard together in a bowl. Season. Arrange kale, chicken and crostini on a plate, drizzle with dressing and sprinkle parmesan over top.

Dinner

WARM SPELT SALAD WITH RADICCHIO, BORLOTTI & TALEGGIO

SERVES: 1
PREPARATION: 5 MINUTES
COOK: 35 MINUTES

1 tablespoon butter
½ small red onion, chopped
80 g (2¾ oz) spelt, rinsed
1 tablespoon white wine
300 ml (10 fl oz) boiling vegetable stock
50 g (1¾ oz) canned borlotti (cranberry) beans, drained and rinsed
½ small radicchio, sliced
25 g (1 oz) Taleggio cheese, chopped

Heat butter in a saucepan over medium heat and cook onion for 3 minutes. Stir in spelt and toast for 1 minute, then add wine and simmer until evaporated. Cook spelt by adding a ladleful of boiling stock at a time and stirring frequently. After 15 minutes, add beans and radicchio and cook for another 5 minutes. Turn off heat, add Taleggio, season, stir and cover pan for 2–3 minutes before eating. Serve.

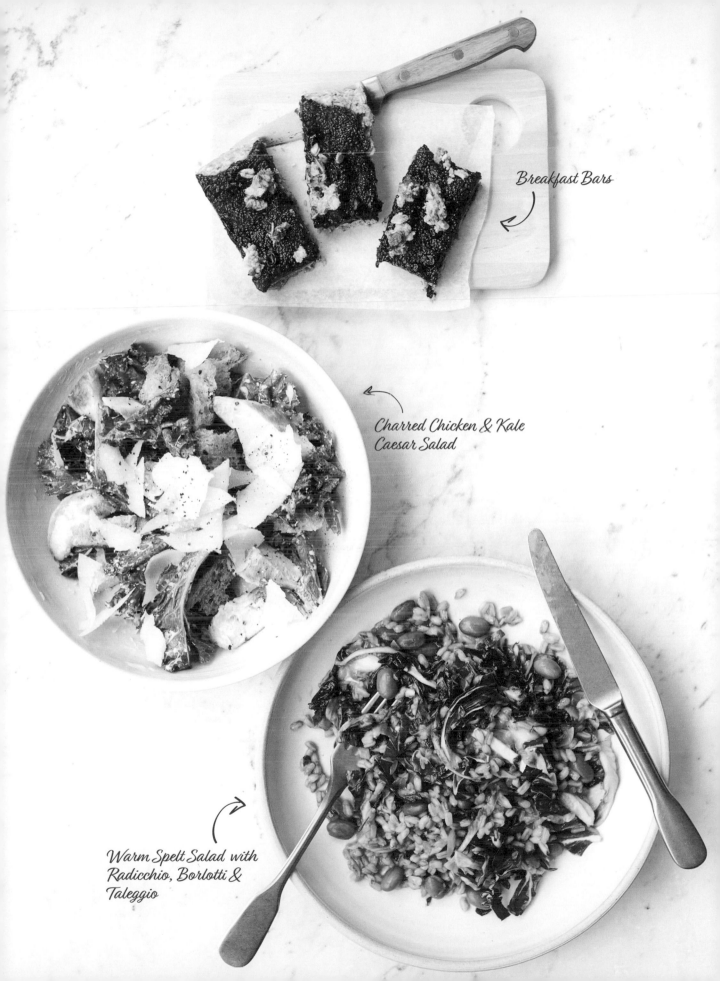

Breakfast Bars

Charred Chicken & Kale
Caesar Salad

Warm Spelt Salad with
Radicchio, Borlotti &
Taleggio

Sunday

This loaf for breakfast is soft, moist and flavoursome. It is also perfect as an afternoon snack. You can store the rest of the soup for lunch in the fridge for another time.

Breakfast

BANANA & MIXED SEED LOAF

SERVES: 1
PREPARATION: 5 MINUTES
COOK: 40 MINUTES

300 g (10½ oz) spelt flour
1 teaspoon baking powder
1 tablespoon dark chocolate chips
200 g (7 oz) mixed seeds
4 bananas, 3 mashed and 1 sliced lengthways
75 g (2¾ oz) caster (superfine) sugar
80 ml (⅓ cup) rapeseed oil
2 eggs, lightly beaten
150 g (5½ oz) Greek yoghurt

Preheat oven to 180°C (350°F). Mix flour, baking powder, chocolate chips and 160 g (5½ oz) mixed seeds together in a large bowl. In another bowl, mix mashed bananas, sugar, oil, eggs and yoghurt together. Add banana mixture to dry ingredients and mix well. Pour into a lined 20 x 10 x 8 cm (8 x 4 x 3¼ in) loaf tin, sprinkle with remaining seeds and put halved banana on top. Bake for 40 minutes, or until a skewer in centre comes out clean. Cool in tin for 5 minutes, then transfer to a wire rack to cool completely. Slice and store for 2–3 days.

Lunch

PROBIOTIC COLD GAZPACHO

SERVES: 2
PREPARATION: 5 MINUTES
COOK: 0 MINUTES

250 g (9 oz) ripe tomatoes, halved, plus diced tomatoes, to garnish
½ red onion, finely diced
½ garlic clove, mashed
1 small cucumber
½ small red bell pepper (capsicum)
1 teaspoon apple cider vinegar
1 tablespoon extra virgin olive oil, plus extra for drizzling
60 ml (¼ cup) kefir milk
salt and pepper

Blitz tomato halves in a blender for 30 seconds. Add remaining ingredients and blitz to a thick and smooth soup. Season and serve, garnished with diced tomatoes and drizzled with oil.

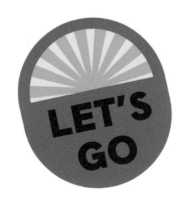

Dinner

CHILLI SALMON NOODLES

SERVES: 1
PREPARATION: 5 MINUTES
COOK: 10 MINUTES

2 tablespoons soy sauce
2 tablespoons mirin
1 teaspoon chilli sauce
1 salmon fillet, skin on
70 g (2½ oz) buckwheat noodles
½ tablespoon sesame seeds
1 spring (green) onion, sliced

Mix soy sauce, mirin and chilli sauce together in a small bowl and use half of mixture to coat salmon. Heat a frying pan over medium heat and cook salmon, skin-side down, for 3 minutes, then turn over and cook for another 1 minute. Remove and keep warm. Meanwhile, cook noodles in a large saucepan of boiling water according to packet instructions and drain well. Lightly toast sesame seeds in frying pan over medium heat for 3 minutes until fragrant, add cooked noodles with remaining sauce and toss to mix. Serve with salmon and spring onion.

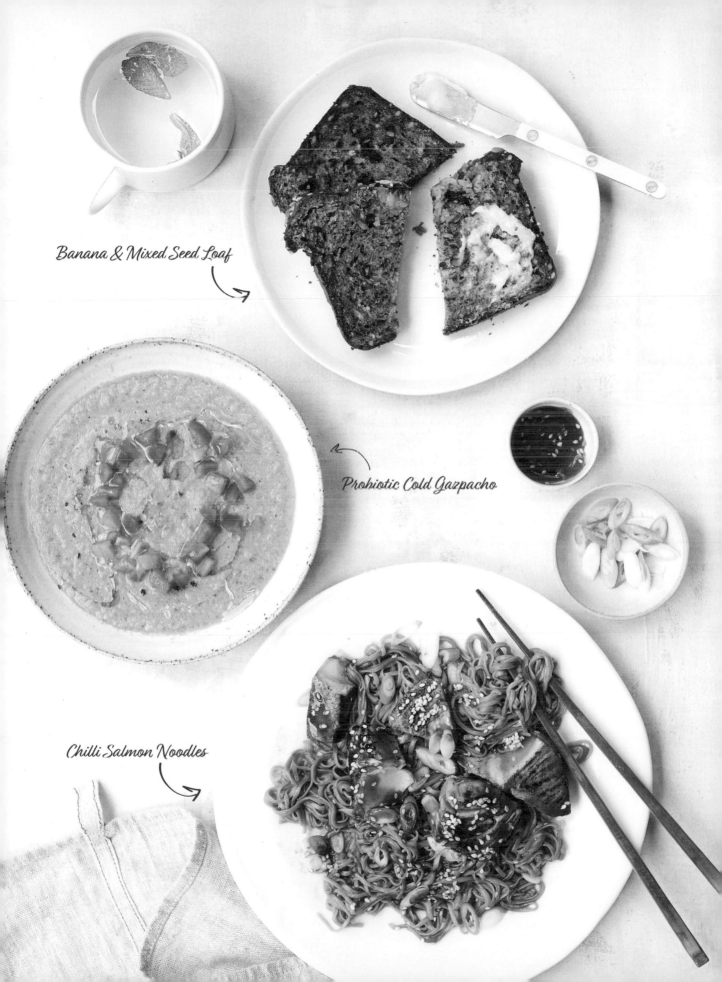

Banana & Mixed Seed Loaf

Probiotic Cold Gazpacho

Chilli Salmon Noodles

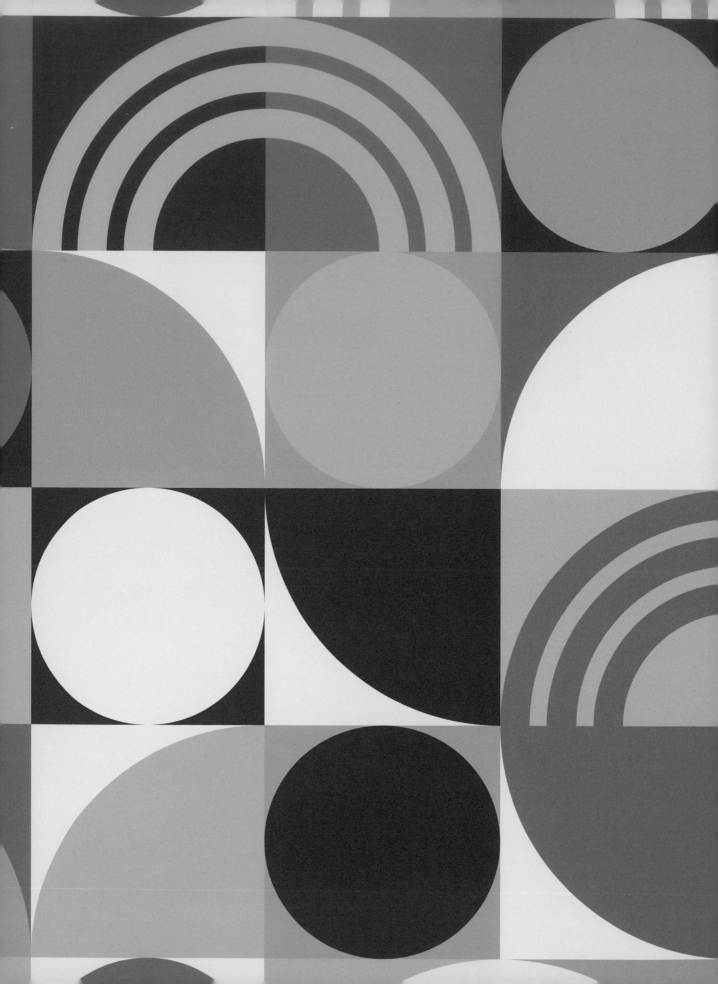

Snacks &
Drinks

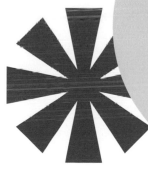

WITH

- Healthy dressings to elevate your dishes to the next level
- Dips to add to your dishes or snack on
- Healthy alternative drinks instead of coffee
- Refreshing tonics that are healthy for your gut

Drinks

Sometimes it is good to alternate coffee with other non-caffeinated drinks. Try kombucha, a mildly fizzy fermented drink, rich in probiotics and antioxidants, or a refreshing tonic made with ginger and turmeric packed with antioxidants that help to cleanse your body and strengthen your immune system.

KOMBUCHA TEA

MAKES: 1 LITRE (4 CUPS)
PREPARATION: 7–14 DAYS
COOK: 5 MINUTES

2 teaspoons loose-leaf black tea
100 g (3½ oz) granulated sugar
1 SCOBY (symbiotic culture
    of bacteria and yeast)

Put leaf tea into a 1.2 litre (41 fl oz) heatproof glass jar. Bring 1 litre (4 cups) water and sugar to the boil in a large saucepan, then pour over the tea, cover with muslin (cheesecloth) and leave overnight. Next day, strain tea into another large jar and add SCOBY. Cover jar with muslin, so SCOBY can breathe, and secure it with an elastic band. Leave to ferment in a warm room out of direct sunlight for about 7–14 days. Try a sample every 2 days until it reaches your desired flavour, then remove SCOBY and 200–250 ml (7–8½ fl oz) starter liquid for next batch. Pour kombucha into sterilised glass bottles and store in fridge. Kombucha is ready to drink immediately or add flavourings, such as fruit, herbs and spices, then ferment for another 2 days in fridge. Use SCOBY for up to a month at room temperature resting in some kombucha.

LEMONGRASS, GINGER & TURMERIC TONIC

MAKES: 250 ML (1 CUP)
PREPARATION: 5 MINUTES
COOK: 10 MINUTES

1 cm (½ in) piece ginger, peeled
½ lemongrass stalk, outer leaves
    removed, halved lengthways
2.5 cm (1 in) piece turmeric root or
    1 tablespoon ground turmeric
splash of tonic water
juice of 1 lemon
½ teaspoon maple syrup
1 slice grapefruit, to serve

Put ginger, lemongrass, turmeric and 250 ml (1 cup) water into a saucepan and simmer for 10 minutes. Strain and leave to cool. Top up with tonic, add lemon juice and maple syrup. Stir and serve cold with grapefruit slice.

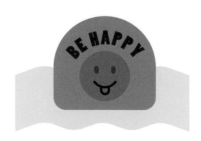

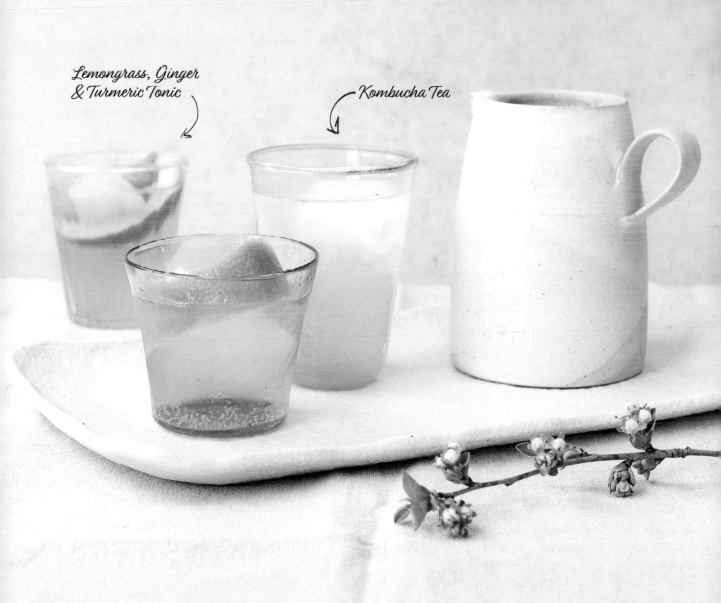

Lemongrass, Ginger & Turmeric Tonic

Kombucha Tea

Snacks

You can be creative with a dipping sauce and elevate your dish to another level, whether it is as a base for a sandwich, a topping on a grain bowl to add extra flavour, or served with some crunchy vegetables or corn chips. Using cannellini beans and lentils, two superfood ingredients filled with prebiotics and fibre, you can easily make a dip or hummus, which is rich in flavour and packed with healthy protein.

BUTTERNUT & RED LENTIL HUMMUS

MAKES: 220 G (8 OZ)
PREPARATION: 5 MINUTES
COOK: 20 MINUTES

70 g (2½ oz) red lentils
100 g (3½ oz) cooked butternut
  squash
½ teaspoon sea salt
1 teaspoon tahini
1 teaspoon chopped coriander
  (cilantro)
2 tablespoons extra virgin olive oil
1 tablespoon lemon juice
salt and pepper

Put lentils into a saucepan, cover with water, bring to the boil then simmer for about 20 minutes, until soft. Drain and put them into a food processor with butternut squash, salt, tahini and coriander and blitz for 1 minute. With machine still running, drizzle in oil and lemon juice and blend to a smooth consistency, adding some water, if needed. Season to taste.

RED PEPPER & HARISSA DIP

MAKES: 200 G (7 OZ)
PREPARATION: 5 MINUTES
COOK: 0 MINUTES

100 g (3½ oz) canned cannellini
  beans, drained and rinsed
70 g (2½ oz) roasted red bell pepper
  (capsicum)
1 tablespoon extra virgin olive oil
1 teaspoon lemon juice
¼ teaspoon chopped coriander
  (cilantro)
1 teaspoon harissa paste
½ garlic clove, chopped
salt and pepper

Put all ingredients into a food processor and pulse until smooth. Season with salt and pepper. Store in an airtight container in fridge for up to 7 days.

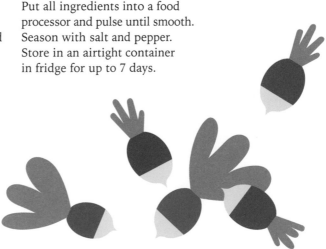

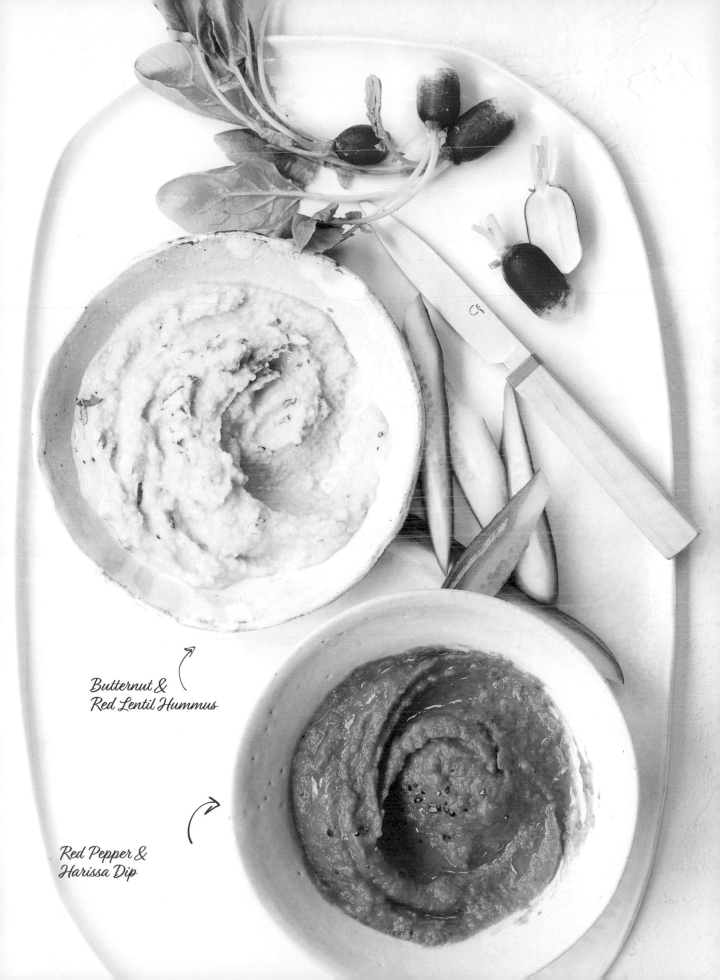

*Butternut &
Red Lentil Hummus*

*Red Pepper &
Harissa Dip*

Dressings

These two dressings are simple to make and are packed with superfood ingredients. Delicious and rich, both these dressings can be added to lots of dishes – use to top grilled, roasted or seared meat or simply toss them into a healthy soup.

SEEDY GREMOLATA

MAKES: 80 G (2¾ OZ)
PREPARATION: 5 MINUTES
COOK: 0 MINUTES

50 g (1¾ oz) mixed pumpkin and
    sunflower seeds, toasted and
    roughly chopped
grated zest of ½ lemon
1 tablespoon chopped parsley
¼ teaspoon chilli flakes
1½ tablespoons extra virgin olive oil
salt and pepper

Mix seeds, lemon zest, parsley, chilli and oil together in a bowl. Season with salt and pepper and serve. Store leftovers in an airtight container for 2 days.

MISO & WALNUT SAUCE

MAKES: 240 ML (8 FL OZ)
PREPARATION: 5 MINUTES
COOK: 10 MINUTES

5 Kalamata olives, pitted and
    roughly chopped
100 ml (3½ fl oz) extra virgin olive oil
75 g (2¾ oz) red miso paste
1 garlic clove, grated
½ teaspoon chilli flakes
50 g (1¾ oz) walnuts, finely chopped

Put olives into a saucepan with oil over low heat. Add miso, garlic and chilli and simmer for 5 minutes, stirring. Stir in walnuts and cook for another 2 minutes. Store in an airtight container in fridge for up to 3 days.

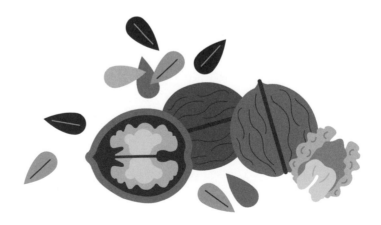

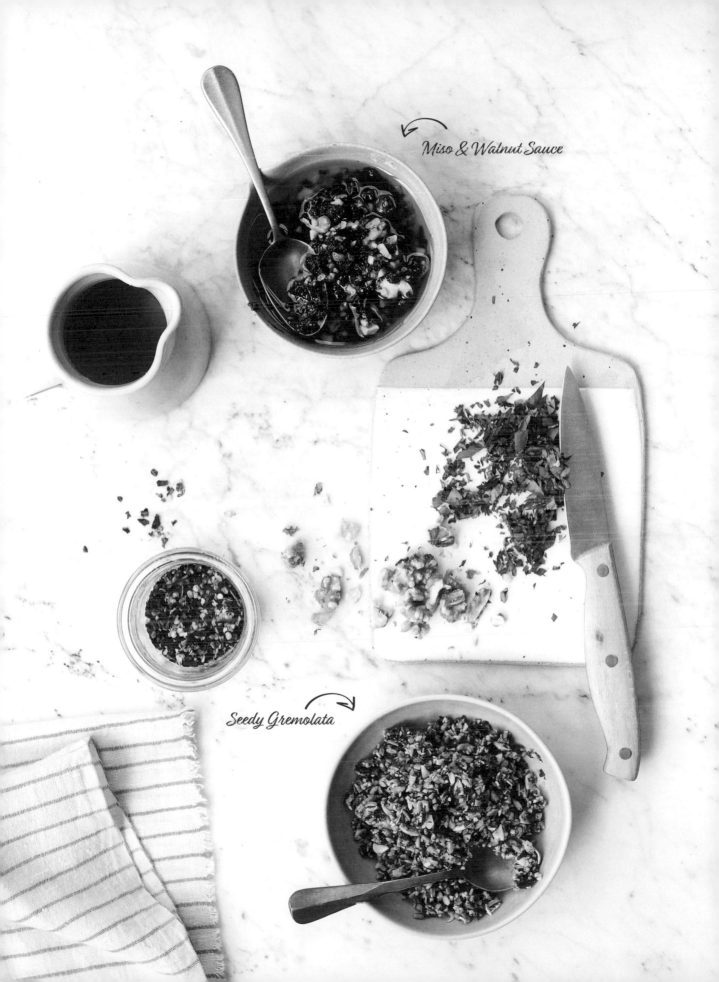

Miso & Walnut Sauce

Seedy Gremolata

Snacks

Deeply savoury and fragrant with seeds, these crackers are a great afternoon snack served with a healthy dip while the delicious combination of oats, seeds and chocolate make these bars, packed with healthy protein and fats, an option all day long.

HIGH-FIBRE DARK CHOCOLATE, OAT & SEED BARS

MAKES: 12
PREPARATION: 5 MINUTES
COOK: 20 MINUTES

150 g (1½ cups) rolled (porridge) oats
100 g (3½ oz) mixed seeds
20 g (¾ oz) pistachios
85 ml (2¾ fl oz) maple syrup
50 g (1¾ oz) dark chocolate chips
2 tablespoons coconut oil, melted

Preheat oven to 160°C (320°F). Lightly blitz oats in food processor, then put into a bowl and add rest of ingredients. Mix, then spread in a lined 20 cm (8 in) square baking tin, pressing down well. Bake for 20 minutes or until golden brown. Cool, then cut into bars. Store in an airtight container for a week.

MIXED SEED CRACKERS

MAKES: 340 G (12 OZ)
PREPARATION: 10 MINUTES
COOK: 20 MINUTES

200 g (7 oz) mixed seeds (sunflower, pumpkin, chia, sesame, linseeds/ flax seeds)
1 teaspoon sea salt
1 tablespoon thyme
2 tablespoons extra virgin olive oil

Preheat oven to 160°C (320°F). Combine mixed seeds, salt and thyme in a large bowl. Add oil and 100 ml (3½ fl oz) water, mix together and leave for 10 minutes until seeds absorb the water. Put the dough onto a lined baking tray and cover with another baking tray. Using a rolling pin, spread dough out thinly, about 3–4 mm (⅛–¼ in). Remove paper and bake for 20 minutes, or until golden brown. Transfer to a wire rack to cool, then break into irregular shards and store in an airtight container for up to a week.

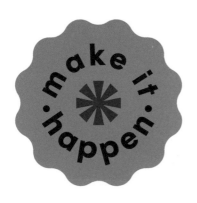

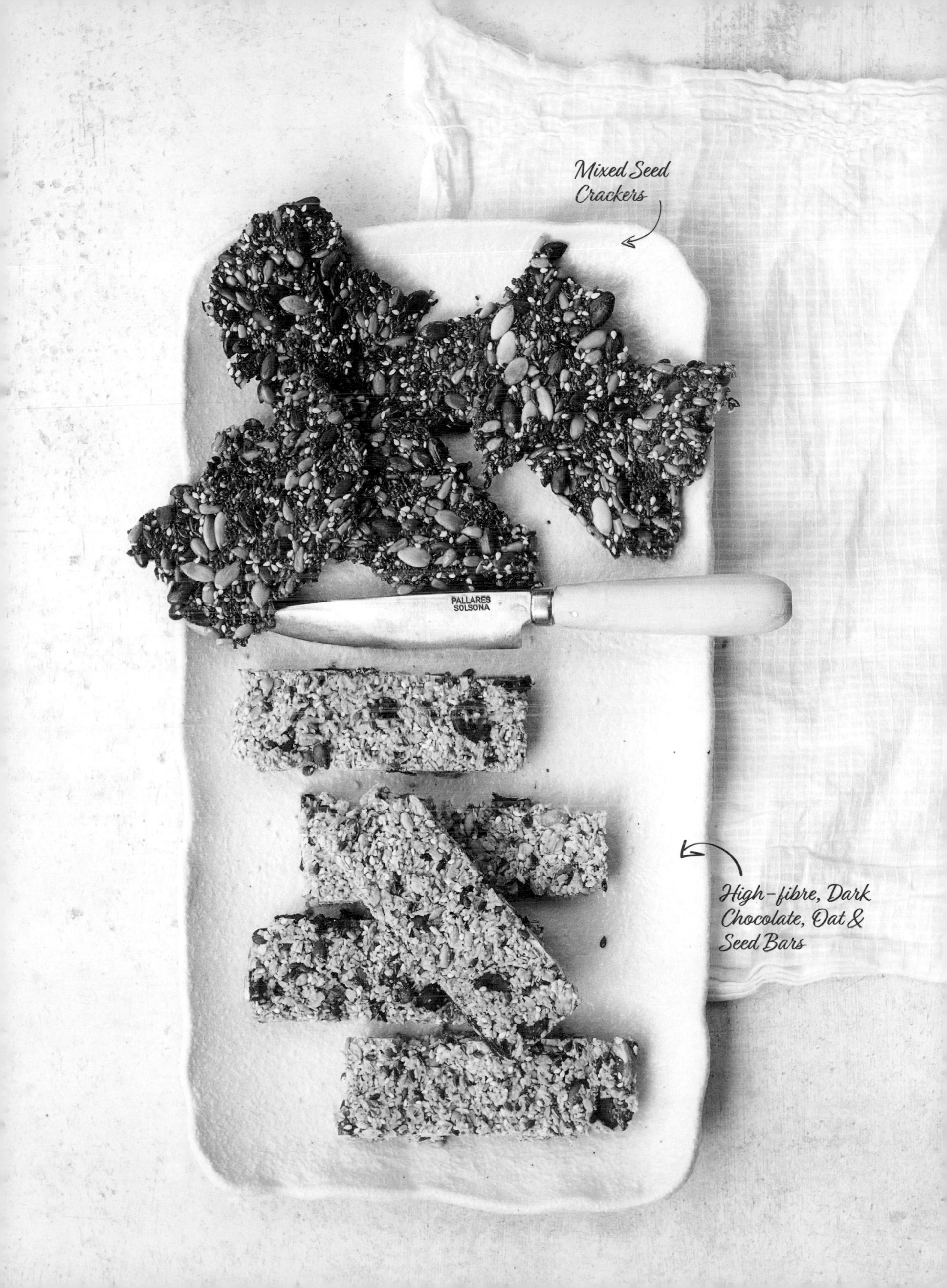

Mixed Seed
Crackers

PALLARES
SOLSONA

High-fibre, Dark
Chocolate, Oat &
Seed Bars

Recipes per week

List of recipes

Dinner

Baked Sweet Potato with Whipped Feta & Sumac	112
Barley, Cannellini, Tomato & Watercress Stew	102
Beef Tacos with Kimchi Sauce	120
Broad Bean Stew	134
Caramelised Roast Cabbage with Lentils	82
Cauliflower Soup	122
Chickpea & Saffron Soup with Live Yoghurt	84
Chilli Salmon Noodles	140
Creamy Mushroom & Taleggio Polenta	80
Gnocchi with Mushroom Ragout	96
Grilled Eggplant & Lentil Salad	114
Lentil & Chickpea Burgers with Cucumber Pickle	132
Marinated Lamb Chops with Couscous Salad	108
Mediterranean Mackerel with Cauliflower Purée	106
Mediterranean Soup	136
Pan-roasted Chicken with Olives, Lemon & Thyme	124
Pan-roasted Chicken with Orange & Olives	88
Pappardelle with Cavolo Nero & Parmesan	86
Provençal Pistou Soup	98
Roast Tomato & Crispy Kale Soup	104
Salmon Fishcakes & Pickle	116
Seafood Paella	100
Spelt & Bean Stew	92
Spicy Fajita Buddha Bowl with Beans	128
Stuffed Peppers with Spelt & Goat's Cheese	118
Sweet Potato & Red Onion Soup	130
Warm Spelt Salad with Radicchio, Borlotti & Taleggio	138
Zucchini Noodles with Ricotta & Basil	90

Drinks & Snacks

Butternut & Red Lentil Hummus	146
High-fibre Dark Chocolate, Oat & Seed Bars	150
Kombucha Tea	144
Lemongrass, Ginger & Turmeric Tonic	144
Miso & Walnut Sauce	148
Mixed Seed Crackers	150
Red Pepper & Harissa Dip	146
Seedy Gremolata	148

Basics

Classic Kimchi	64
Lacto-fermented Pickles	74
Live Yoghurt	66
Sprouting Seeds & Pulses	68
Super Seedy & Multigrain Granola	72
Triple Nut Butter	70

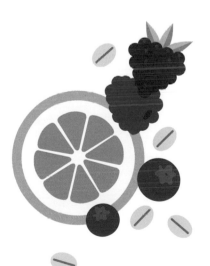

Index

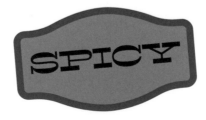

Index continued

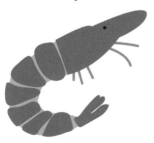

ACKNOWLEDGEMENTS

Clémence Cleave

Thank you to Catie, the publisher, and all the team at Marabout, for trusting me in writing a compelling and instructive book about gut health! To Giovanna, my co-author, for creating so many delicious gut-friendly dishes. To Kathy, Frankie, Lisa and Michelle for bringing the text to life with stunning pictures and great illustrations. To Chris for his encouragement and careful proofreading. And finally to all the nutrition scientists and researchers who keep revealing more and more secrets of this inner-world that is the gut – a truly fascinating field!

Giovanna Torrico

A huge thank you to Catie Ziller who gave Clémence and me the opportunity to write this book. It was a really exciting challenge but it was made easier thanks to the knowledge and experience of Clémence, thank you! Always grateful to the magic team: Frankie, Lisa, Michelle and Kathy and to my husband, Salvatore, and my children, Luca, Mario and Andrea.

BIOGRAPHIES

Clémence Cleave (MSc, Clinical Nutrition – ANutr) is a nutritionist, a trained chef and a visiting lecturer in nutrition science at the University of Roehampton, London. Born in France, she lives in London with her family where she practises as a coach and consultant nutritionist. Her expertise is in women's health, weight management, disordered eating behaviours and gut health. She writes books and articles, runs workshops and coaches groups and individuals to enable people to find their unique and optimal diet, and improve their health behaviours and well-being.

Giovanna Torrico was born in southern Italy, where she inherited a deep passion for food. She is a pastry chef and caterer based in London, UK. Her books include **Cake Decorating Step by Step**, **Italian Bowls**, **The Zero Waste Cookbook** and **Clean Cakes**.

First published in French by Hachette Livre, Marabout division
58, rue Jean-Bleuzen, 92178 Vanves Cedex, France

This edition published in 2023 by Smith Street Books
Naarm | Melbourne | Australia | smithstreetbooks.com

ISBN: 978-1-92275-4-158

Publisher: Paul McNally
Editor: Ariana Klepac
Internal designer: Michelle Tilly
Cover designer: Murray Batten
Photographer: Lisa Linder
Stylist: Frankie Unsworth

Printed & bound in China by C&C Offset Printing Co., Ltd.

Book 246
10 9 8 7 6 5 4 3 2 1

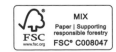

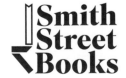